People With Diabetes Can Eat Anything

It's All About Balance

Jane K. Dickinson, RN, PhD, CDE

Published by Media 117

Table of Contents

Mom, I know how you can get rid of diabetes.
Take your kit and all your diabetes stuff and say,
'I'm not going to do this anymore.' And then
throw away all the stuff in your office and say,
'I'm getting a different job.'
My son at age five

Mom, what's a weird activity you like to do?
Oh, I know one: counting carbs!
My daughter at age ten

Introduction

I live and work with diabetes every day: I have type 1 diabetes, and I am a health care professional working with patients who have diabetes. I hope to use my personal and professional experience to benefit you, the reader. Although my personal experience is with type 1 diabetes and insulin, far more people have type 2 diabetes, and the messages in this book are for everyone. Some parts may not apply to you, for instance, if you don't take medication or if you don't use insulin. You can either skip those sections, or read along and learn something extra! This book is written for people with diabetes and just as much for people without diabetes. I often get calls from family members or friends of people with diabetes: "My friend/cousin/mother-in-law is coming to town, she/he has diabetes, and I need to know what kind of food to have in the house." I hope this book will be helpful to those people as well. I also want to provide information to those who are at risk for diabetes. I hope you never get it. Regardless of why you chose this book, all readers are invited to visit my website, www.janekdickinson.com, and let me hear from you!

My main purpose for writing this book is to help readers achieve a healthy relationship with food and feel empowered to manage their diabetes successfully. I hope to answer the question that almost all patients with newly diagnosed diabetes, many people who have had diabetes for years, and their family members ask as soon as they enter my office: *What can I eat?* The answer I give every one of those people is the same: *People with diabetes can eat anything.* I hope readers will come away from this book understanding and believing that *it's all about choices* and that they are truly *your choices to make.* Whether you choose to eat only plant-based foods, or you are a meat lover; whether you eat whole grains or low carb, it's about being informed and figuring out what works best for you and your body. It's about owning your disease, feeling good, having energy, and getting on with your life. I also hope to help readers *without* diabetes gain an understanding of what it's like to live (and eat) with diabetes, and become more informed about how it all works. According to the 2011 Centers for Disease Control (CDC) statistics, approximately 26 million Americans have diabetes and an additional 79 million have pre-diabetes (1); these numbers are increasing every day! This means that many, many people need to get the message, and preferably right away. People with diabetes make up about eight percent of the American population, and I strongly believe that the other 92 percent needs to hear the message too.

I was diagnosed with diabetes at a time when the disease was managed very differently than it is today. In some ways, being told you had diabetes was like being handed a prison sentence: we were told we had to take medications at certain times and eat certain foods at certain times – every day for the rest of our lives. Luckily, we've come a long way since the 1970s. If you still feel like you're in prison, it's time to break free!

Diabetes was named by a Greek physician in the first century A.D. The disease has not changed, but our understanding of it, philosophy toward it and management of it are drastically different. Diabetes has gone through name changes as well. Once referred to as Insulin-Dependent (Type I or Juvenile Onset) and Non Insulin-Dependent (Type II or Adult Onset) Diabetes Mellitus, we now call it type 1 or type 2 diabetes. Although the most important thing is just to know that you have diabetes, it makes sense to know what type of diabetes you have. I believe that knowledge is power: the more you know, the more powerful you are in your ability to take care of yourself. The fact that you are reading this book shows that you care about learning more about your diabetes and your health. I also believe that you are in charge of your own health. You are the most important person on your health care team, and you are responsible for understanding and managing your diabetes.

Type 1 diabetes is an autoimmune disorder in which the body turns on itself and kills off the cells in the pancreas that produce insulin. With type 2 diabetes, people still produce insulin; however, their bodies do not use it properly and/or they do not make enough. It is important to know what type of diabetes you have so you can be sure you are managing it properly. It's also helpful when explaining your condition to others. Aside from potential differences in medications (and their side effects), the basic principles of managing type 1 and type 2 diabetes are the same. This book is for people with both type 1 and type 2 diabetes. There is a third type of diabetes called gestational diabetes mellitus or GDM. This type of diabetes can occur in women who are pregnant. Despite my battle cry of "people with diabetes can eat anything," which I will repeat often in these pages, I will mention that for women with gestational diabetes (and women with pre-existing diabetes who are pregnant) it is simply easier and safer to manage diabetes during the pregnancy if certain foods and drinks are avoided. There is a special note on this in Chapter 2 and a section in Chapter 9.

Diabetes is a very complex disease that has an impact on just about every aspect of health and the human body. Scientists continue to study and learn more about diabetes every day. Because my goal is not to duplicate efforts that have already been made, I have addressed, but not gone into great detail, on a number of diabetes-related topics in this book. There are countless resources available where you can learn more about these topics; I have made recommendations for further reading throughout the book. All of these books are also listed in the Appendix. In addition, ask your health care provider for reliable diabetes resources. I will mention several times in the pages ahead that although the Internet is a wonderful and convenient way to gather information, be wary of what you read. Stick with websites that are sponsored by the government (".gov") or an academic institution (".edu"). There are also several non-profit organizations that provide reliable information on the Internet (".org"). Diabetes social networks are helpful for many people; be sure to double check what you learn with your health care provider, and remember that everyone's experience with diabetes is unique.

Diabetes has been around for thousands of years, but people have only been *living* with diabetes for less than one hundred years. Before that people were dying from diabetes. In this day and age, we don't have to die from diabetes. There is so much that we know about diabetes and how to manage it in order to live successfully with the disease. Unfortunately, somewhere along the line, diabetes became equated with the statement, "you can't eat sugar." This is simply not true.

Not only health care professionals, but people with diabetes themselves and the general public have contributed to perpetuating this message. And the message of what people can and cannot eat leads to blame and shame and a very negative attitude toward a disease that can be very manageable.

Carbohydrate is the type of nutrient that breaks down into glucose (sugar in the blood) the fastest in the human body. Even though we know that carbohydrate is the most important (and efficient) energy source, negative messages about carbohydrate have been circulating for the past several years. Throughout the book I use the terms, "carbohydrate," "carb," and "CHO" interchangeably. If I use "carbohydrates" or "carbs" (plural), I am referring to carbohydrate servings. We'll dive further into this carbohydrate topic than you ever cared to in Chapters 2 and 3, but for now to expand on my earlier answer: *People with diabetes can eat anything, as long as they pay attention to how much, how often and how it affects their blood glucose (sugar).* Sound simple? Well, it's not. But it doesn't have to be as complicated or as dismal as it is often made out to be.

Diabetes is one of the most common diagnoses in the world right now. People are better off finding a way to live successfully with it, or we'll end up having a world full of miserable and/or sickly people. We have no control over how long we'll be here on earth. What we do have some degree of control over is the quality of our lives while we're here. Paying attention does not necessarily mean weighing and measuring food: it means living a balanced life and feeling good about the choices we make. It means knowing that we are doing the best we can and in doing so, achieving the results we want.

Food plays a large role in our culture, and sometimes in religious practices. Because it is impossible to address every existing culture or religion in the context of this book, I have only used basic examples. It is important for people with diabetes to work with a health care professional to find ways to incorporate cultural and religious practices into their diabetes management and vice versa.

As a professional educator I feel compelled to help others live successfully with diabetes, and I am convinced that people with diabetes use three things to do so:

1. a positive attitude
2. ownership
3. choices

I'm a big believer in balance, as well, and I think balance is the result of having a positive attitude, owning our diabetes, and making choices. For as long as I can remember, people have used the term "balance" to describe diabetes management. For many years it was balancing medication, exercise, and food. We've added stress management and other items along the way. Ultimately we don't just need balance in diabetes management, but in life, and diabetes management is just one part of our lives. Diabetes involves a lifelong learning process, and there are resources available to help shape our attitude, take care of our bodies, and make healthy choices each day. Confidence is also an important tool for managing diabetes successfully. With accurate, up-to-date knowledge, we can build our confidence and live a healthy life with diabetes.

In the past several years a lot has happened in terms of diabetes and food: fad diets have come and gone, and research has revealed new information about nutrition. The more we learn about food, "diets," and nutrition, however, the more it seems that a simple and straight-forward approach is best. What you'll find in the pages that follow are stories, thoughts and explanations of a simple and straight-forward approach to living with and managing diabetes.

You will notice that there are some things I repeat (even several times) in this book. This is most likely because I feel it's important and deserves emphasis. You will also notice that frequently throughout the book I suggest consulting with your health care provider. The value of finding a health care provider who is a good fit cannot be overstated.

This book does not claim to have a "cure" for diabetes, nor is it a weight-loss plan. My goal is to help readers find in themselves the motivation to make healthy choices, and an understanding that their attitude will drive their outcomes. This book is not meant to be a "how-to," but more of a guiding, supporting and informing resource. In every chapter you will notice sections called "Tasty Morsel (of information)," which provide extra tidbits of information and "A little exercise," which are do-on-your-own practice activities. Feel free to write in the book (unless you borrowed it from a friend or library or it's an e-version) or complete these exercises on a separate piece of paper.

This book is based on principles of my philosophy that people with diabetes can eat anything. Just as there is a lot more to diabetes than food, that statement really means more than just food. One could cut out the "eat" and replace it with a number of other words ("pursue," "accomplish," "achieve," etc.). This book, above all else, is meant to set people with diabetes free from the burden of thinking they are limited in any way and clear up the message to the world. Bon appetit!

Chapter 1
I Have Diabetes: Now What?

I've never taken well to being told I can't do something.
30-something male with type 1 diabetes

I was diagnosed with type 1 diabetes at the age of seven. I went from being a high-energy first grader who chased boys on the playground and played "Froggy Baby" with my best friend, Jenny, to sitting in the shade playing Barbies® at recess. My teachers told my parents something was wrong. I went from running around the neighborhood after school to sitting on the couch and watching television. My mother knew something was wrong. I peed all the time and got very thin. My father knew something was wrong. I remember many times on car trips when I made the family wait because I had to use the bathroom…***again***. Grandpa told me many years later that they all thought I was dying.

After school was over for the year, I ended up in the hospital. Originally I was taken to the pediatrician who diagnosed me with a bladder infection and prescribed antibiotics, which did not work. After a week I wasn't getting better so we returned to the pediatrician's office and this time he told my mother that I had diabetes and needed to go to the hospital. When we left the office, my mother took me to Friendly's (an ice cream shop headquartered in Massachusetts) and said I could have whatever I wanted for being so good, so I ordered up a strawberry milkshake. While this was *not* a typical response from my mother, it was a little foreshadowing of my mother's diabetes wisdom. In other words, she did not freak out and tell me I could *never have ice cream again*. Of course, she may not have known exactly what was going on yet, either.

To those of us who live with it, diabetes may seem like the most common, everyday thing imaginable. However, some people are diagnosed with diabetes and know absolutely nothing about it. Perhaps they only know what they've heard from friends or relatives. There are a lot of misconceptions about diabetes lurking around out there (starting with "you can't eat *xyz*," but we'll get to that in just a minute). I once met a patient who was in her 40s and newly diagnosed with type 1 diabetes. She was baffled at how she could possibly have diabetes when she runs marathons, eats nutritious foods and generally lives a healthy lifestyle. Unfortunately, type 1 diabetes can happen anytime – and so can type 2. This patient's boyfriend was very frustrated with the choices of books on diabetes. "Why isn't there a book that says, 'This is a manageable disease; you can still live a long, productive and healthy life with diabetes'?" I assured him that I was working on it!

It is incredibly important for a person's experience at diagnosis to go well. Whether someone feels intimidated, judged, accepted, or empowered when they are diagnosed with diabetes can make or break their experience with the disease. If you are reading this book shortly after being diagnosed, take advantage of the information in these pages and develop the best attitude toward diabetes that you possibly can – it will pay off! If you have already had diabetes for a while or even a very long time, you can still adjust your attitude and have better outcomes, so keep reading! Sometimes people are told they have type 2 diabetes when they actually have type 1 diabetes. A good example of this is Zippora Karz, a professional ballerina who wrote the book, *The Sugarless Plum*. In the case of my 40-something patient above, the health care professional gave her the correct diagnosis; however, she did not know enough about diabetes to understand that it had nothing to do with how much she exercised, or what she ate.

> **Tasty Morsel (of information):** If you lost weight without trying, drank fluids incessantly, and went to the bathroom frequently (including overnight) before being diagnosed, you could actually have type 1 or LADA (latent autoimmune diabetes in adults). LADA is sometimes called type 1.5 diabetes. If this is the case, you likely need to take insulin (and not diabetes pills). Check with your health care provider to clarify or confirm your diabetes diagnosis.

After being diagnosed with diabetes, most people living with the disease will tell you the hardest part is food. The food thing can definitely be a challenge. Sure, it would be great if we could just cut out high-fat, high-calorie foods (or whatever our "vice" happens to be), and some people have that ability. But not everyone. So the rest of us need to find a way to have a healthy relationship with food. It is possible to quit smoking or drinking alcohol "cold turkey." But we can't quit eating. We must have food to survive for any length of time. At one time, food was just that – a means of survival. Food was not necessarily connected to comfort or romance or reward. That has evolved over many years. Another thing that evolved was the "thrifty gene." This is something humans developed in order to survive periods when food was scarce. Nowadays, since food is plentiful, the "thrifty gene" just contributes to obesity.

> **Tasty morsel (of information):** In 1962, geneticist James V. Neel first described the idea of the "thrifty gene" (2), suggesting that certain human genes have

evolved to promote fat storage. This was beneficial during times of scarcity; however, due to the current abundance of food and sedentary lifestyles, these genes now lead to obesity and diabetes. This is not an excuse for type 2 diabetes, but very possibly a contributing factor.

Not only is food plentiful, but unhealthy food is readily available and often cheaper, while healthy food can be more expensive and harder to find. Wouldn't it be wonderful if everyone could have a garden in their backyard? I really think it would be the answer to many of our problems. Instead we depend on produce stands or grocery stores for our fruits and vegetables, but sometimes the cost is overwhelming or even prohibitive.

It has been noted that if you go to the grocery store and stay only on the perimeter of the store, you will find the freshest, most healthy food choices. The aisles in the middle are loaded with processed, packaged, high-fat foods. Is this true where you shop? Take notice next time you are there. In many ways our lives have become ruled by convenience. Because we work so hard, we want to buy something quick and easy for a meal. This often means the packaged stuff in the middle of the store. I, for one, buy frozen lasagna instead of making my own.

Fast food has been getting a bad rap for years, but what factors lead people to eat fast food? It's cheap, it's fast and it's convenient. The high fat content makes it taste good too. The American dream is more for less, right? At fast food places we get just that. And the more we get the less we benefit. The purpose of this book is not to chastise people for being overweight, nor to criticize Americans for making unhealthy choices that are so easy to make. The purpose of this book is to help people with diabetes, those who love them, and the general public to see that it is, indeed, all about choices.

When patients with diabetes walk into my office and ask, "What can I eat?" or when they say, "Tell me what I can and can't eat" or even, "Tell me what he/she (meaning their spouse/mother/father) can and can't eat," I look them in the eye and respond: "Anything."

People with diabetes can eat anything.

And everything people with diabetes put in their mouths potentially affects their blood glucose. It's simply a matter of how much, how often and how the food affects blood glucose levels. Ok, so it's not *simple*, but it's also not the prison sentence that was once laid down on any person with diabetes.

Historically, when someone was diagnosed with diabetes, they were told to take certain amounts of certain medications at certain times. They were also often told they were never to eat sweets again. They were instructed to follow a strict "diabetic diet." In fact, when I was diagnosed with type 1 diabetes at age seven, I was put on a 2200-calorie "diet," which no one ever changed or adjusted as I grew older, taller, went through puberty, pregnancy, etc. I'd like to clear up a few things. There is no such thing as a "diabetic diet." The message for people with diabetes is the same as it is for the general public: *eat healthy, well-balanced meals; everything in moderation; consume whole grains, fruits and vegetables, low-fat dairy and limit saturated and trans-fats.*

In defense of those who promoted the "diabetic diet" for many years, we need to understand its origins. Before we knew much about diabetes, and certainly before we had insulin and other medications, people with diabetes were put on a "starvation diet," which consisted of very little to no carbohydrate. Our forebears knew that diabetes was a problem with carbohydrate metabolism, and they figured out that if people with diabetes followed a high fat/low carb diet, they could prolong life – for a while.

> **Tasty Morsel (of information)**: Here is an excerpt from a book published in 1916, *The Starvation Treatment of Diabetes*: "For forty-eight hours after admission to the hospital the patient is kept on ordinary diet, to determine the severity of his diabetes. Then he is starved, and no food allowed save whiskey and black coffee. The whiskey is given in the coffee: 1 ounce of whiskey every two hours, from 7 a.m. until 7 p.m. This furnishes roughly about 800 calories. The whiskey is not an essential part of the treatment; it merely furnishes a few calories and keeps the patient more comfortable while he is being starved" (3).

Once insulin was discovered in the early 1920s (a wonderful book to read is called *The Discovery of Insulin* by Michael Bliss), people were no longer starved as a diabetes treatment. Instead, patients were told to consume high-fat foods, protein and some carbohydrate. For a while everyone was convinced that insulin was a cure, so no one emphasized healthy eating habits. Over time it became obvious that people with diabetes had a very high rate of heart disease, and the "diet" wasn't helping. In 1971 came the "ADA Diet" (American Diabetes Association). This was an eating plan that prescribed a certain number of calories per day, broken into "exchanges." The ADA put out a booklet of "exchange lists," which placed food into six categories: milk, meat, starch, fruit, vegetables and fat. At that point, patients were being told how much and when they "could" eat. Over time, professionals began to realize that high-fat meal plans were not healthy and encouraged slightly more carbohydrate and less fat; however, the damage had been done.

People with diabetes, their friends, family, society at large and many, if not most, health care professionals believed with all their hearts that people with diabetes cannot eat sugar. And this is the message that has been passed down from generation to generation.

Back in the days before insulin was available, the majority of people with diabetes had type 1 diabetes. Type 1 diabetes is an autoimmune disease in which the body produces antibodies that attack and kill off the cells in the pancreas that make insulin. People cannot survive without insulin, because insulin is responsible for transporting glucose from the blood into the cells, where it is used to make energy. Over the years, however, type 2 diabetes has become more and more prevalent. Type 2 diabetes is characterized by insulin resistance, a situation where the body does not efficiently use the insulin that it makes, or insulin insufficiency, where the body does not make enough insulin. The body still produces some insulin in type 2 diabetes, and people can live with high blood glucose levels for many years. Over time, however, people with type 2 diabetes typically produce less and less insulin. During this time of not enough insulin working (or being produced), damage can occur to blood vessels all over the body.

Today, the rates of type 2 diabetes are significantly higher than type 1 diabetes: at any given time approximately 90-95% of all people in the United States who have diabetes, have type 2 diabetes. When this book was being written, about 26 million Americans had diabetes (that's about 8% of the population), and this number is growing all the time. In addition, about 79 million Americans have pre-diabetes (1). Pre-diabetes means that the fasting blood glucose level is elevated, but not quite high enough to be considered type 2 diabetes. People with pre-diabetes can make lifestyle changes to prevent getting full-blown type 2 diabetes;

however, left alone, pre-diabetes will progress to type 2 diabetes in a matter of time.

Latent autoimmune diabetes in adults (LADA) is yet another form of diabetes mellitus with subtle differences from both type 1 and type 2. In fact, LADA appears to have similarities to both types 1 and 2, yet does not completely fall in either category. Some people call it type 1.5 diabetes. People with LADA are typically diagnosed during adulthood. They may manage with pills for a short time (typically less than six years) and then require insulin. Often they do not require a lot of insulin to meet their needs. People with LADA are often diagnosed with type 2 diabetes first, because of their age and because they respond to oral medication (at first). They are often thin at diagnosis and experience elevated blood glucose levels, weight loss, thirst and frequent urination.

> **Tasty Morsel (of information):** The only definitive way to know what type of diabetes someone has is to perform a blood test. If someone has positive *insulin auto-antibodies*, it is definitely type 1 diabetes. Insulin auto-antibodies attack the cells that make insulin and cause someone to stop making insulin. A blood test called a "C-peptide" test can also be measured, which determines whether someone is still producing insulin. Insulin starts out as pro-insulin, which contains a c-peptide chain and an insulin chain. C-peptide breaks off and insulin goes to work. People with type 2 diabetes typically test positive for C-peptide since they produce insulin. Because LADA has a slower onset than type 1 diabetes, these patients may have a positive C-peptide at first, which could be misleading.

Some people don't get much more or better information now than people did years ago. I can't tell you how many people I talk to who swear they were never told they have diabetes. Communication gaps may exist between what health care providers say (and how they say it) and what patients hear. No one wants to hear a diagnosis of diabetes, so if what they heard was "your blood glucose is high and you need to start taking this medication," they may not think they actually have diabetes. Another thing I encounter a lot in patients is fear. Some people, when told they have diabetes, can think only of the great aunt who died from diabetes complications or the friend who "can't eat anything." Some people are fearful because they honestly don't know anything about diabetes. All too often patients say, "I'm scared to eat." *My hope for you, the reader, is that any fears you have about food and diabetes will be relieved as you read this book.* Fear doesn't lead us to positive outcomes; rather it bogs us down, and being afraid of food is just a downward spiral. Confidence and knowledge are the tools that help us overcome fears and start on the path to health and happiness. As I've mentioned, this book is about choices, and you get to choose whether or not to be fearful.

Over the years, and as the result of many research studies, we have come to know that people with all types of diabetes *can* metabolize carbohydrate, as long as there is a balance of food, insulin (medications) and activity. Since 1994, the message of nutrition management and diabetes has been, "a carb is a carb is a carb." This means that it does not matter so much what the carbohydrate source: as long as the amount of carbohydrate is the same (in grams), the effect on the blood glucose is ultimately the same. And, of course, healthy carb choices in healthy amounts are better for us in the long run.

> **Tasty Morsel (of information)**: In 1994 the American Diabetes Association publicized its position that when the same amount of carbohydrate is consumed, despite the source (for example, an apple vs. a brownie), the blood

glucose effect is the same. At that time, the American Diabetes Association began promoting a meal plan that contains moderate amounts of sugar, doing away with a "diabetic diet." All these years later, we still hear people (even health care professionals) say that "people with diabetes can't eat sugar," which simply is not true (4).

Getting back to the "people with diabetes can eat anything" message. Literally, people with diabetes, just like people without diabetes, can – *have the ability to and have the choice to* – eat anything. People with diabetes, unfortunately, have gotten dragged down in this feeling that they are *not allowed to* eat just anything. Although well-meaning, those who did and still perpetuate the message that people with diabetes can't eat certain things, often do more harm than good. Health care professionals who promote the idea that people with diabetes can't eat certain foods only set up an environment of shame, blame, failure and judgment. That's really not fun for anyone. Spouses and other family members who watch over shoulders and "remind" people with diabetes not to eat certain things are seen only as nags, which is yet another downward cycle. When I asked my sister (who was nine when I was diagnosed) what she experienced at my diagnosis, she said she felt she had to make sure I didn't eat anything with sugar in it. She claims she was not told she had to do this, but she just felt it was what she was supposed to do. Interesting.

It is important, actually crucial, that we take on the food thing. We need to understand how to handle food and then carry it out with confidence and conviction. That way the rest of the world can only say, "Wow. She/he really knows what she/he is doing with diabetes." I can't even tell you how many times I have heard family members or friends of people with diabetes say, "So and so just eats whatever he/she wants and then takes a bunch of insulin." This leads the general public to believe not only that people with diabetes can't eat certain things, but that they are a bunch of reckless sloths who do it anyway. I don't know about you, but I don't want to be lumped in with that crowd. I encourage you to take really good care of yourself and eat well *most* of the time. When you do choose to indulge – do it with style and grace, confidence and care. And enjoy!

Earlier I mentioned that despite being able to (and allowed to) eat anything, paying attention to how much, how often and how it affects our blood glucose can keep us healthy. Some approaches we can try when dealing with the how much part are eating smaller portions, eating fewer sweets and junk foods, and eating consistent amounts from day to day. When dealing with the how often part we can work on eating at least three times a day, and eating at consistent times from day to day. We'll discuss these ideas more in future chapters. As far as how it affects the blood glucose, this is determined by checking blood glucose levels, and there is an entire chapter dedicated to this topic later on.

It is important to note that just as there are many people living with diabetes, there are many different ways people manage their disease – especially the food part of it. There are countless meal plans out there; the important thing is to get the nutrients your body needs so you stay healthy, feel good, and have energy to lead a productive (and fun) life. And it's always good to remember that what works for one person may not work for another.

Younger kids with diabetes, whose parents provide three healthy meals each day, at relatively the same times, are probably the only group who don't have trouble with the "how often" part of this. Eating three meals a day may not be a big deal if you're a kid and your parents are providing and preparing all the food (this may also be the case for some adults). Many families make healthy food choices, in terms of how much and how often they eat. Many parents are aware of the long-term effects of high-fat foods, partially hydrogenated oils (trans-fats), and so on. But others are not. Kids with diabetes are at the mercy of those who put the food in front of them (or put the food in the refrigerator and on the shelves). If you are a parent of a child with diabetes and you are reading this book, chances are you already do or are planning to make healthy choices for your family – for that you deserve credit!

Parents can make sure there are no "forbidden foods." This approach helps to avoid developing in children a feeling of deprivation and a subconscious need to overindulge in "treats" later on. As long as the message has always been "you can eat anything" and that is done in a healthy, balanced way, kids are less likely to rebel and/or become closet eaters. Small children need help making healthy food choices, whether or not they have diabetes. It is important for kids with diabetes to learn about things like candy, cookies, etc., and how they affect the blood glucose and health in general. My kids constantly ask me, "Is (fill in the type of food/beverage) good for you?" And I always answer, "Not if you eat it all the time, every day. If you eat it once in a while, it's ok." There are some exceptions. When they ask about things like apples, I explain that if we ate apples all the time, every day, they would still be good for us, but we need other types of food to get all the nutrients our bodies require to be healthy and strong.

In a perfect world, families would have healthy eating habits. Being handed a diagnosis of diabetes in their child, despite causing sadness for many reasons, would not mean having to change anything in terms of the meals and snacks served at home. Unfortunately, people often assume that diabetes means they're doing something wrong and they have to change. Diabetes is equated with restriction and limitations. Diabetes makes people think "good" and "bad." The mother of an 11-year-old boy with newly diagnosed type 1 diabetes asked me, "What are some good snacks?" My explanation was that snacks are not good or bad. Some snacks are healthier than others, and some can raise the blood glucose level more or faster than others. Therefore, the family and/or the person with diabetes needs to use the information that they have (how their blood glucose responds to the food, how they feel after they eat it) to determine whether or not they want to eat it, how much of it they want to eat, or how often. Let's take Reese's® peanut butter cups® as an example. I love Reese's® peanut butter cups®. I know that two standard peanut butter cups equal a carb serving (15 grams of CHO) and for me require one unit of insulin. I know that peanut butter cups are a high-fat food item. I also know that if I overeat peanut butter cups it's hard to manage my blood glucose and I usually don't feel good physically. As a result, I choose not to make eating peanut butter cups a regular part of my life. Every now and then, however, I will enjoy a peanut butter cup (or two). I have even found dark chocolate and organic peanut butter cups. Even better!

The majority of people with diabetes are adults, however, and adults are typically on their own when it comes to eating. It can be hard to stick to the "three squares" we grew up on when dealing with all the responsibilities of adulthood. Work, parenting and other activities often take precedence over healthy eating. As a result, many adults with diabetes find themselves with pretty erratic eating patterns. This can affect all three: how much, how often, and how it affects the blood glucose.

Many people find it rare that they eat a healthy breakfast, a healthy lunch and a healthy dinner. More often, they skip breakfast or eat something from a convenience store or coffee shop for breakfast, like a bagel or a muffin. They might eat this item at some point during their morning work hours. Maybe they end up skipping lunch or they grab a snack (again a convenience or fast-food item), and come home ravenous at the end of the day. This may or may not describe you. On the other hand, people who eat healthy meals and exercise can sometimes still get diabetes. Some people really don't need to change much in the way they are eating. If you feel that you already make healthy food choices and get regular exercise, but your blood glucose is not responding, you may need a different type or amount of medication. That's something to discuss with your health care provider.

> **Tasty Morsel (of information):** It is generally believed that apple-shaped (android) bodies, where extra fat accumulates in the abdomen, are at higher risk for diabetes. Pear-shaped (gynoid) bodies, where extra fat accumulates in the hips, buttocks and thighs, are not. This means that people who carry extra weight around their middle (apple shape), even if they are otherwise thin, have a greater chance of getting type 2 diabetes. People who carry extra weight in the abdomen typically have fat tissue surrounding their vital organs. Although it was thought that these people had a higher risk for heart disease, research is now showing that obesity, in general, puts people at higher risk of heart disease (5).

Because people with diabetes were led to believe – for a very long time – that they can't eat certain foods, the general public has also gotten this idea engrained in their heads. In fact, anyone can benefit from following the same principles that are taught to people with diabetes. There is no difference in nutrition recommendations for people with and people without diabetes. Once again, *everything in moderation; whole grains; high fiber; low-fat dairy; fruits and vegetables, lean or plant-based protein, and limited saturated and trans-fats for all!* Some of you are still not convinced. You're thinking: "but something has to be different for people with diabetes, or they wouldn't be told they have the disease." You're right. What's different is that people with diabetes have more responsibility. Everything they put in their mouths potentially affects their blood glucose. We'll go over this in much greater detail in future chapters, so read on.

Some of you are reading this and thinking, "You are wrong! I can't eat _____ (fill in the blank – cheesecake, cooked carrots, pasta, mashed potatoes, brownies, or whatever). It makes my blood sugar go through the roof!" I would ask you to pause for a few moments and think about *can* vs. *choose*. I truly believe that attitude goes a long way. If you have a healthy, positive attitude you will have better outcomes. First and right away, you will feel happier. Second, and over the long run, your health will improve, or be maintained. People who consider diabetes a prison sentence get what they asked for – imprisoned. They are chained by dietary *rules* and they succumb to the food police. These people tend to say, "I can't," or "I shouldn't" a lot. People who approach diabetes as an opportunity (ok, that may be stretching it a bit), or at least something that is doable, tend to have an easier time managing it. These people tend to take ownership and say, "I won't," or "I don't want to." This is a choice.

> **Tasty Morsel (of information):** When I think about being positive, I don't mean irrational or delusional – expecting things that aren't realistic or even possible. By positive I mean engagement, enthusiasm, excitement – creating an environment that leads us to achieve what we are after and having good outcomes. Being positive is

changing the things we can and for everything else, changing the way we look at it; think about it; approach it.

The gentleman quoted at the beginning of the chapter was referring to anyone implying that there were things he can't do because of diabetes. This young man is very active outdoors, and his activities have not changed since he acquired diabetes. His quote is also appropriate regarding food. Being told we *can't* eat something often just makes us want it more. By owning our diabetes and managing it through our choices, we feel empowered and strong. When we allow ourselves to feel imprisoned, we become weak and lose sight of those choices. I suggest keeping our eyes open and only looking forward. For kids with diabetes, parents can help them own it: help them see that it's all about choices and that their lives can be full, productive and positive, even with diabetes onboard.

My goal is to be independent in managing my diabetes. I meet with my endocrinologist (physician who specializes in diabetes) periodically to check in, find out the latest and greatest, ask questions, and make adjustments to my management plan as needed. I find that I learn something new every time I go. There is always something new to learn about diabetes – even if you've had it for many, many years! I have the same goal for those I work with professionally. I want each of them to feel confident in managing their diabetes independently. All of us need to know how to manage our choices in terms of how much, how often and how they affect our blood glucose levels. I consider myself a resource, support person and cheerleader, but not a crutch. My hope for you, the reader, is that you will come away from this book feeling that you've learned something, knowing that you can manage your diabetes successfully, and knowing how to use your resources. Of course, I also want you to know that living a healthy, abundant life with diabetes is not only possible, it's your choice.

Chapter 2
The Food Thing

Yes, I can eat that. Often, I probably shouldn't. But neither should you.
40-something female with type 1 diabetes

Despite my strong feeling that *there is more to diabetes than food*, this book promises to address *the food thing*, so here goes. Please keep in mind, as you read the following two food chapters, that food is not the focus of this book. The focus is attitude, choices, and living well with diabetes. So when I write that *people with diabetes can eat anything*, I mean that what you choose to eat is literally that – *your choice*. I believe that people with diabetes can follow all sorts of meal plans – whatever works best for the individual – and that it's more important to eat with a healthy attitude than follow a particular "diet." If you are angry and frustrated about eating certain foods, it's really not going to do you any good. These chapters are simply meant to provide some background information on food and meal plans so you can make informed choices. Reading about food, thinking about food, and eating food has become a source of anxiety for many people. My goal is to help you overcome those feelings and enjoy your meals.

When I was diagnosed with type 1 diabetes, I was immediately placed on a 2200 calorie "diet." My dad created a "meal plan card" based on what my parents were taught at the hospital, and this "card" hung inside a cabinet door in my parents' kitchen for years. In fact, it was still there after I finished college and went out on my own. At one point, my dad wrapped it in plastic to preserve it, and it no longer hangs on that door (I've checked), but I'm sure he's got it somewhere. Back then the thinking was that since people with diabetes can't metabolize carbohydrate, just fill them up on fat. That was a throw-back from the days of starving people with diabetes to keep them alive (see Chapter 1). When I was sent to diabetes camp to learn how to give insulin injections, I was forced to eat crazy amounts of fat at every meal. One time I had a couple pats of butter and a wad of peanut butter left on my plate. My counselor said I had to eat it all. She sat at the table with me until I did. I can't stand the sight of peanut butter and butter on the same knife, let alone eat them together, to this day!

> **Tasty Morsel (of information):** I could write another entire book on the benefits of diabetes camp. The truth is, I didn't think it was so great as a kid in the 70s, when they were force-feeding me fat and making me learn how to give my own injections. However, diabetes camp has changed and adapted over time, and they don't use scary tactics in the dining hall anymore. And kids learn how to give their injections when they are ready. I strongly encourage children and adults to give diabetes camp a try; there are all sorts of programs available. If you are too old to be a camper, consider being a staff member, and there's always family camp. In fact, there's something for everyone. Find out about a diabetes camp program near you by visiting the Diabetes Education and Camping Association's website: www.diabetescamps.org.

Of course, what we know about food in general, and the food/diabetes connection is growing and changing all the time. Today there are theories that high-fat and low carb meal plans are healthy for some people (more on that later) and we know that plant based fats have healthy qualities.

I was once giving a talk on diabetes for the health care and daycare providers of a very young boy with type 1 diabetes. At one point, a nurse practitioner piped up and asked, "Why don't you just tell him, 'You can't eat sugar'?" It doesn't make sense to just make a blanket statement like, "You can't eat sugar" for several reasons: 1) it's not nice, 2) it could backfire, and 3) it's not true! People with diabetes *can* eat sugar. They (or their caregivers in this situation) just need to know how to handle it. It turned out that the woman who suggested we tell this child "you can't have sugar" has a child with food allergies. On a regular basis she told her child, "you can't eat that" because, indeed, if her child ate certain things he/she could die. While eating certain things in excess can cause health problems, people with diabetes learn to make choices by understanding how foods will affect them and the possible outcomes of eating them. In my experience, people who make informed choices are happier and more successful than those who are forced or guilted into action.

Believe it or not, there is "sugar" in many of the foods we eat! Fruit, for example, is one of the healthiest foods available, and fruit has "sugar" in it. People with diabetes learn how to incorporate fruit into their daily eating plan by eating the appropriate amount, taking the appropriate medication(s), and/or exercising after eating it. Since 1994, we have used "carbohydrate" rather than "sugar" to describe sweet or starchy foods. This includes grains, cereals, crackers, rice, pasta, cakes, cookies, fruit, starchy vegetables and milk, which are all carbohydrate-containing foods. Sweetened drinks also contain carbohydrate. There are numerous types of sugars and they are all carbohydrate. We know that the same amount of carbohydrate has approximately the same affect on a person's blood glucose level, regardless of its source; therefore, it is now conventional to refer to "carbohydrate" ("CHO" or "carb") rather than "sugar."

Carbohydrate

The food we eat is made up of three types of nutrients: carbohydrate, protein and fat. We call these three "macronutrients" because they are needed by the body in large quantities. Vitamins and minerals, which are needed only in small quantities, are called "micronutrients." In the world of diabetes, we often focus on foods that affect the blood glucose level. Carbohydrate (carb) has the biggest and fastest effect on the blood glucose level. Carbohydrate gets broken down and starts turning into glucose in the body within about twenty minutes of eating, which raises the blood glucose. Carbohydrate foods can be sugary (simple carbohydrate) like cakes, cookies, candy and fruit, or starchy (complex carbohydrate) like potatoes, pasta, grains and rice.

Carbohydrate is a good source of energy for the human body. We often think of carbohydrate as "brain food": the human brain needs glucose to function, and the brain is in charge of the rest of the body, so we don't want to deprive it. There are also eating approaches that target fat as brain food, which works for many people who choose a low carb lifestyle. The human body breaks down carbohydrate efficiently to form glucose, which then fuels the brain and the rest of the body. Fat can also be broken down to make energy, but using a different process. There are different thoughts about how much carbohydrate each person needs. For many years the message has been that most people need 45% to 55% of their daily caloric intake from healthy carbohydrate foods. But for many people this message is changing. When we do eat carbs, the important thing is to figure out the right amount for our body and to choose healthy carbs. Healthy carbohydrate sources include whole grains (high fiber), fruits and vegetables, and low-fat dairy. Below is a partial list of healthy carbohydrate foods.

- Brown rice
- Whole grain pasta
- Whole grain bread
- Beans (black beans, pinto beans)
- Potatoes (with skin)
- Other starchy vegetables like beets, carrots, peas, winter squashes, corn
- Fat-free milk
- Low-fat yogurt
- Fruit

I have met with several patients who report being told that they should stay away from fruit, or that fruit is "bad." Fruit is not bad. Fruit is a natural, healthy source of carbohydrate. Fruit is loaded with vitamins and minerals that our bodies need. However, fruit also has a significant effect on blood glucose levels. Fruit will raise the blood glucose relatively fast, and there are ways to handle that.

In the early 1990s people started using an approach to nutrition management of diabetes called "carb counting." This was about the time that nutrition scientists announced that "a carb is a carb is a carb," meaning that all carbohydrate has the same basic effect on blood glucose. It also became common knowledge that people with diabetes can eat sugar as long as it is worked into the management plan in a safe and healthy way. Carb counting means counting the grams of carbohydrate about to be eaten and calculating the amount of insulin needed to help metabolize that carbohydrate (keep the blood glucose in the target range). The "carb ratio" or "insulin-to-carb ratio" is the amount (in grams) of carbohydrate that one unit of insulin covers. This varies from person to person. It is best to work with a diabetes health professional to calculate your insulin-to-carb ratio, if you use one.

Carb counting has revolutionized nutrition management of diabetes because no longer do we take a certain amount of insulin and then eat a certain amount of food. Carb counting allows us freedom in our food choices and amounts. There are some unfortunate consequences of carb counting, however, including potentially eating too much. Some people have a tendency to overeat carbohydrate foods and take lots of insulin to "cover" it. This can lead to weight gain. Another drawback is overlooking protein and fat. Because we don't "count" protein or fat in this approach, some people eat too much protein and fat, and others don't eat enough. *The goal of any eating plan in managing diabetes is to eat healthy foods in healthy amounts in order to keep blood glucose levels as close to normal as possible.*

There are excellent lists of foods and their carbohydrate content available. The *Exchange Lists for Diabetes*, published by the American Diabetes Association in cooperation with the American Dietetic Association, is an excellent resource. It is also very simple to find carbohydrate lists online. If you do a quick search for "carbohydrate content of ..." many options will come up. Another helpful American Diabetes Association publication is *The Complete Guide to Carbohydrate Counting* by Hope Warshaw and Karmeen Kulkarni.

The rule of thumb is that 15 grams of carbohydrate is one "carbohydrate serving." If you look at one of these lists, you can determine how much of your favorite fruit one serving equals. If you are not counting carbs as part of your diabetes management plan, knowing the size of a carbohydrate serving can still serve as a point of reference.

Tasty Morsel (of information): The typical carbohydrate requirement for a non-pregnant adult is at least 130 grams per day. On average, women eat 3 to 4 carbohydrate servings (45 to 60 grams) per meal, and men eat 4 to 5 servings (60 to 75 grams). This is a starting point, and these recommendations will vary based on height and weight, age, weight loss goals, activity level, etc. If you are unsure of how much food you need for your ideal weight, make an appointment to see a registered dietitian. For those who are following a low carb lifestyle, these numbers will vary greatly.

What about potatoes? Potatoes have taken a beating in the last several years, but potatoes are not the enemy. Remember, everything – including potatoes – in moderation. It is true that, like fruit, potatoes raise the blood glucose level. It is also true that eliminating carbohydrates from your food choices can lead to weight loss – even rapid weight loss. Over the years, many people who lose weight by following a low carb meal plan put the weight back on, and some put on additional weight as soon as they resume eating carbohydrate. There are many people who have found success managing their diabetes by drastically cutting back on carbohydrate, while many others find it difficult to live without carbohydrate (6). The key is to add healthy carbs in moderation and find a good balance where healthy weight, blood glucose, and lipid levels can be maintained. Some people find it works best to stay low carb for the long haul, while others can add a little more carb to their meal plan.

Healthy carbohydrate choices, when eaten in the right amounts, do not lead to weight gain. Some people find they are better off avoiding potatoes (and that is their choice) due to elevated post-meal blood glucose levels, but many people who include potatoes as part of a healthy meal plan, do just fine.

Protein

Most people think of "meat" when they think of protein. Beef, pork, chicken, and turkey are all examples of protein. Other types of protein include fish, eggs, tofu, and dairy products. Protein can also be found in vegetables and other plant products such as beans, lentils and nuts. Protein is an important nutrient because it plays several critical roles in our bodies, but people sometimes think we need more protein than we do.

Proteins, which are made up of chains of amino acids, help with support, movement, transport, buffering, metabolic regulation, coordination and control, and defense in the human body. Enzymes, hormones, and antibodies are proteins. Although protein is a very important nutrient, it doesn't take a lot to meet our bodies' needs. One serving of protein is one ounce, or seven grams, which looks like the size of a deck of cards or the palm of your hand. The recommended intake of protein is only up to 20% of what we eat, so it's easy to overeat protein.

Too much protein can lead to problems, because often we tend to eat high calorie foods such as a half-pound burger with cheese, or a steak). Many of these foods – depending on their source and how/whether they are processed, can be less healthy for us. And these choices can lead to weight gain. When choosing protein, you can make it healthy by opting for lean cuts of meat, grass-fed beef, poultry, fish, or plant-based proteins. Eggs are fine in moderation for most eating plans. Check with your health care provider if you have questions about eggs. Some people choose to follow higher protein meal plans. Again, it's all about what works best for you in terms of health blood glucose levels, feeling good, and achieving healthy outcomes.

Fat

In the "old days," the meal plan actually dictated how many servings of fat we were to eat at each meal. When we finally figured out that people with diabetes do not necessarily need to avoid carbohydrate and consume high-fat "diets," we went through a phase where "low fat" was in. Now we know that balance is best and that there are some fats that are more healthy than others. Trans-fats are not healthy; they come from refined carbs or processed foods. Trans-fats are found in packaged foods such as chips, crackers, cakes, and cookies. There are varying thoughts on saturated fats, which are the ones that mostly come from animals. Examples of saturated fats include butter and cream and foods that are made with butter and cream.

Monounsaturated and polyunsaturated fats are healthier. They come from plants: nuts, olives, olive oil, avocadoes, peanut or other nut butters. Omega-3 fatty acids come from fish and other dietary sources and are a very healthy unsaturated fat. Many people take omega-3 fatty acid supplements, but it is possible to get enough from your food. Talk to your health care professional if you are not sure you are getting enough. Here are some sources of omega-3 fatty acids:

- Cold water, oily fish (salmon, mackerel, herring, anchovies, sardines)
- Kiwifruit and some berries
- Flax
- Some nuts (walnuts and butternuts)
- Eggs produced by chickens fed certain diets
- Meat, milk and cheese from grass-fed animals

Oils fall in the fat category, and there are more and less healthy oils. Oils that are either mono- or polyunsaturated fats are better for our heart health. Monounsaturated fats help lower LDL ("bad" cholesterol) without affecting HDL ("good" cholesterol); polyunsaturated fats help lower LDL, but may also lower HDL. The following is a list of healthy oils:

- Almond Oil (monounsaturated)
- Avocado Oil (monounsaturated)
- Canola Oil (monounsaturated)
- Corn Oil (polyunsaturated)
- Flaxseed Oil (polyunsaturated)
- Grapeseed Oil (polyunsaturated)
- Olive Oil (monounsaturated)
- Peanut Oil (monounsaturated)
- Safflower Oil (polyunsaturated)
- Soybean Oil (polyunsaturated)
- Sunflower Oil (polyunsaturated)
- Walnut Oil (polyunsaturated)

Trans-fats are "partially hydrogenated oils," which are oils that have been chemically changed so they will keep foods fresh longer. In other words, trans-fats increase the shelf-life of foods and are found in processed foods. This is why you hear the recommendation, "buy foods from the perimeter of the grocery store," which is where the fresh, whole foods are located.

> **Tasty morsel (of information):** Eating too many saturated fats can increase your triglycerides (stored fats) and LDL. Trans-fats lead to heart disease and may be even worse for us than saturated fats, therefore, making changes in your food choices can lower your triglyceride and LDL levels. The most effective way to raise your HDL is to have a healthy lifestyle: exercise, don't smoke, lose weight (if you need to), eat healthy fats, and

drink alcohol in moderation. Some medications that lower LDL also help raise HDL.

If you have questions about the types of fat you eat, make an appointment to meet with a registered dietitian, who can give you suggestions for how to incorporate healthy fats and limit unhealthy ones in your daily meal plan.

The goal is to find a healthy balance in your eating habits. Choose healthy carbs, healthy proteins, and healthy fats in amounts that maintain a healthy weight and healthy blood glucose levels. Protein and fat take much longer to break down in the body, and they do not turn into glucose as readily as carbohydrate. While some claim that protein and fat do not affect the blood glucose at all, you can decide for yourself, based on how your blood glucose responds. Protein and fat can help prevent glucose spikes after meals, if food is eaten in combination. While eating a food that is pure carbohydrate (for example, an apple or some grapes) would send the blood glucose up immediately, combining the fruit with a handful of nuts or a spoonful of nut butter helps level out the blood glucose after eating.

The downside to protein and fat is that if they are eaten in large amounts, and in combination with high-carb foods, they work to sustain elevated blood glucose levels for several hours. Examples of high-carb/high-fat meals include Mexican-American food often found in chain restaurants (tortilla chips, deep-fried and cheesy items, refried beans), pizza (the crust is carbohydrate; the cheese, oils, and many toppings are fat), and Chinese-American restaurant food (noodles, rice and sauces are high in carbohydrate; oils and added fat are often hidden). You are the expert on your body: do a little "research" and see how your blood glucose responds to protein and fat by checking your blood glucose before and after different meals.

Fiber

It is likely that you've heard about fiber. Lots of people talk about fiber – mostly health care professionals. Fiber is the indigestible part of plant foods. Fiber is emphasized as part of a healthy meal plan for everyone. If you eat a healthy balance of whole fruits, vegetables and whole grains, you are most likely getting enough fiber.

There are two types of fiber: soluble and insoluble. Soluble fiber helps carry fatty substances out of the body, therefore it helps lower LDL. Soluble fiber also plays a role in regulating blood glucose and making us feel full (so we don't overeat). Insoluble fiber helps get food through the digestive tract efficiently and prevents constipation. Fiber can help protect us against cancer and heart disease.

- **Sources of soluble fiber:** cucumbers, celery, carrots, oatmeal, oat cereal, lentils, apples, oranges, pears, oat bran, strawberries, nuts, flaxseeds, beans, dried peas, blueberries, and psyllium.
- **Sources of insoluble fiber:** zucchini, celery, broccoli, cabbage, onions, tomatoes, whole wheat, whole grains, wheat bran, corn bran, seeds, nuts, barley, couscous, brown rice, and bulgur.

The recommended daily intake of fiber is about 25 grams (a little less for women and a little more for men). Beans are a wonderful source of fiber and can be worked into many meals or recipes. The skin of fruits and vegetables often contain the most fiber – be sure to eat the skin of a baked potato or an apple. Whole fruits are encouraged over fruit juice because juice is just perfectly healthy pieces of fruit that have been beaten to a pulp (pun intended). When there is no fiber left, blood glucose rises rapidly after you drink it. By the way, this is the reason that juice is so effective for treating low blood glucose!

Vegetables

Michael Pollan has written several great books about food. We could all live by his quote, "Eat food. Not too much. Mostly plants." Have you heard of the "plate method" for determining what kinds and how much food to eat? You take a plate (circle) and divide it in half. One half of the plate is covered with vegetables. Then you split the other half in half and fill one with whole grains (healthy carbohydrate) and the other with lean protein. This is a healthy meal. You can also add some fruit and healthy fats/oils to round it out. The US government has changed from promoting a "food pyramid" to a food plate. You can find more nutrition information at www.choosemyplate.gov.

I am constantly telling my kids that vegetables are the healthiest and most important food for our bodies. Vegetables are full of vitamins and minerals that serve many purposes and keep us energized and healthy. There are a few "vegetables," like potatoes, sweet potatoes, and corn, that are not really considered vegetables in the diabetes world (so I put them in quotes). Because these vegetables are starchy and raise the blood glucose like carbohydrate, for our purposes they are considered carbohydrate. Peas and carrots can also be considered "starchy" vegetables. Both these vegetables have varying effects on people; for some, they aren't a problem, but for others, they can have a bigger effect on the blood glucose. When I was pregnant, carrots of any sort raised my blood glucose significantly. When I am not pregnant, I can eat several raw carrot sticks without any effect on my blood glucose. Do your own experimenting (eat carrots and check your blood glucose) to find out how you are affected!

Tasty Morsel (of information): Back in the 70s, we referred to "A" and "B" vegetables. "A" vegetables were the ones that did not have that much of an effect on blood glucose, such as green beans, broccoli, and lettuce, while "B" vegetables were the ones that were more starchy (but not as starchy as corn and potatoes), such as peas, beets and carrots. My dad, being a corny guy (no pun intended), would always raise the bowl of peas and say, "does anyone need a P vegetable?"

A little exercise...

Keep a "food diary" for three days. Write down every single thing you eat/drink during that time. You can take this information to a registered dietitian and have them analyze it. You can also analyze it yourself by going to www.choosemyplate.gov and clicking on "supertracker."

Artificial (Non-nutritive) Sweeteners

Non-nutritive sweeteners – sugar substitutes or artificial sweeteners – are those substances that take the place of sucrose (table sugar). They are used in beverages and other food products. After years of research, the evidence shows that these substances are safe and effective in lowering caloric intake, if used properly. Examples of non-nutritive sweeteners include saccharin, aspartame, acesulfame-potassium, sucralose, and stevia, which are described in more detail below.

Saccharin was first discovered in 1879. Saccharin is 300 times sweeter than sucrose, calorie-free and heat stable. Although there was once a concern about saccharin causing cancer, it is recognized as safe. Aspartame is 160-220 times sweeter than sucrose, essentially non-caloric, and breaks down (loses its sweetness) at high heat. Acesulfame-potassium (ACE-K) is 200 times sweeter than sucrose, non-caloric and heat stable. It has a bitter taste, so it is usually blended with another sweetener. Sucralose is made from sucrose, but does not raise blood glucose, insulin levels, or A1C. It is 600 times sweeter than sucrose, non-caloric and heat stable. Stevia is a naturally occurring, plant-based sweetener that is 300 times sweeter than sucrose and essentially non-caloric. Stevia is stable at high heat.

The most important thing to keep in mind when consuming food products sweetened with one of these non-nutritive sweeteners is not to use them as an excuse to eat more calories. In other words, some people have a tendency to eat more "diet" foods, because they mistakenly think that these foods won't affect their blood glucose or their weight. In reality, overindulging in any foods will lead to weight gain. For the most part, foods that contain non-nutritive sweeteners still contain calories from carbohydrate and sometimes from fat and protein too. It is important to read food labels and know what you are getting.

I have been known to tell patients to stick with the "real thing" in moderation. Think about ice cream: real ice cream has carbohydrate and fat. Fat-free ice cream has a higher carbohydrate content. Low carb or "sugar-free" ice cream has a higher fat content. I can't imagine what fat-free, sugar-free ice cream tastes like, so I say go for the real thing in moderation. Of course, if you like the taste of fat-free, sugar-free ice cream, by all means, save yourself the calories and enjoy!

There were some studies that showed people who drink "diet" beverages tend to eat more calories. Some people believed that consuming non-nutritive sweetened foods/beverages triggered overeating for a variety of reasons. Now we are finding that this is not necessarily true. Again, there is the danger of people tricking themselves into thinking they can eat all they want because they are drinking "diet" soda, etc., but otherwise, there is probably no physiological connection between "diet" soda and overeating. I have a photo of myself and some college friends eating all sorts of high-calorie foods and washing it down with Diet Coke®. We used to joke that the Diet Coke® washed away the calories. Not so much.

There are guidelines for how much non-nutritive sweetener we can safely consume; however, the amounts are hard to surpass in a typical person's diet. If you consume crazy amounts of "diet" beverages that are sweetened with non-nutritive sweeteners, you may want to check the current guidelines, which are called Acceptable Daily Intakes.

Nutritive Sweeteners

Sugar alcohols fall into the "nutritive sweeteners" category, because they do actually contribute calories to a food item. They are used in what some people call "dietetic" foods, because they typically provide only half the calories of a sugar-sweetened equivalent. The following is a list of sugar alcohols:

- Xylitol
- Maltitol
- Sorbitol
- Erythritol
- Isomalt
- Lactitol
- Mannitol

While these sweeteners can be used safely, foods made with sugar alcohols still contain carbohydrate, which needs to be counted in the meal plan.

Functional Foods

Functional foods are whole foods or modified foods that contain components believed to provide health benefits. Examples of health benefits include reduced risk of diseases beyond the usual benefits of that food item. Functional foods naturally contain – or have added by the manufacturer - substances that have biological activity in the body. These foods may also be called "superfoods," and they are grouped as follows:

- *Phytochemicals* give foods taste, texture, color and smell; they also have the potential ability to alter health. Many phytochemicals are antioxidants.

- *Antioxidants* prevent damage to the body by oxidation, a process that produces "free radicals" or "reactive oxygen species." The normal processes of breathing and breaking down food to make energy produce free radicals. We increase the amount of free radicals in our bodies by engaging in other activities like sun exposure and eating unhealthy food choices. (Examples of antioxidants include blueberries, red wine, peanuts, grapes, tomatoes, and spinach.)

- *Flavonoids* are another phytochemical found in plant foods. Flavonoids have a role in reducing inflammatory processes such as those that lead to heart disease and type 2 diabetes. (Examples include nuts, red wine, dark chocolate, whole grains, and grapes.)

- *Viscous soluble fiber* (see earlier section on fiber) can reduce the risk of cardiovascular disease when eaten as part of a meal plan that is low in saturated fat and cholesterol. (Examples include barley, oatmeal, and psyllium.)

Since diabetes increases a person's risk for heart disease, it may be worth looking into consuming these heart-healthy foods. What we know about food, however, is constantly changing. It is important to find current and reputable information when making decisions about what to put in your body.

Sodium

Sodium is an important substance because it plays a role in many vital processes that occur in our bodies. Some people mistakenly think that sodium affects blood glucose levels, which it doesn't. Although a sodium deficiency would be dangerous to us, there is no known human "diet" that lacks sodium. On the other hand, too much sodium can lead to high blood pressure, heart disease and stroke, which are diseases for which people with diabetes are already at higher risk. High blood pressure and diabetes tend to go together and both increase the risk of strokes. Therefore, being careful not to overdo sodium intake is important. If you don't use "table salt," that is a step in the right direction; however, people get way more sodium in packaged (processed) foods than they do from salt added in cooking or at the table. Check the sodium content on the nutrition facts label of the next packaged food you buy (or are about to buy). While many food manufacturers are getting onboard with cutting sodium content, we can make conscious choices to lower sodium intake by how we prepare foods and what we buy (see USDA sodium recommendations later in this chapter).

> **Tasty Morsel (of information):** There is a meal plan called the "DASH diet" that can lower blood pressure by helping people to decrease their sodium intake and increase activity levels. DASH stands for Dietary Approaches to Stop Hypertension. People who follow the "DASH diet" increase their intakes of potassium-rich fruits and vegetables, eat nuts, fish, whole grains and low-fat dairy products. Things like red meat, butter and other high-fat foods are eaten occasionally. Following this "diet" can help prevent or lower high blood pressure.

Alcohol

Many people have one or two alcoholic beverages several days a week, and in moderation, there is nothing wrong with drinking alcohol. In fact, the recommendation for people with diabetes is 1-2 drinks per day. There are some reported benefits to drinking alcohol, specifically red wine (7). Red wine contains a flavonoid, called resveratrol, that has been shown to fight disease. People who drink red wine may have less risk of developing cancer, heart disease and heart attacks. However, the amount of resveratrol in red wine may not be enough to protect us. Talk to your health care provider about whether you would benefit from a supplement that contains resveratrol.

Here's what I tell my patients about alcohol: "It goes in like carb and is stored like fat." Alcohol is often referred to as "empty calories," because it has no nutritional value. I was once told by an eye doctor, "If you don't drink alcohol, don't start now." And I once met a patient who was diagnosed with type 2 diabetes and told by her physician (at the same sitting) that she had to start drinking red wine every day. Talk about mixed messages! I'm guessing my eye doctor is not a drinker and this patient's physician is.

There are definitely drawbacks to drinking alcohol in excess. As I already mentioned, alcohol is stored as fat, which means excess weight. It usually goes directly to the abdomen, increasing the risk for type 2 diabetes. If you already have type 2 diabetes, adding abdominal fat can increase your resistance to insulin and make your diabetes that much harder to manage. This also means increased risk for heart disease, and drinking alcohol in excess puts people at risk for liver disease as well. Drinking alcohol can affect your ability to think and function clearly, which can lead to accidents, poor performance at work, relationship problems, and difficulty managing diabetes. Excessive intake of alcohol damages the organs of the body. Elevated blood glucose damages the organs of the body. So if you put the two together, you're not doing your body any favors.

People who take insulin have a higher risk for low blood glucose (see Chapter 8) when they drink alcohol. Because the liver is busy breaking down the alcohol, it can't help out by sending glucose when someone becomes low. This effect, coupled with being "drunk," can put someone in real danger. Someone who is drunk may not recognize that they are low because the signs and symptoms of being drunk and being low can often mimic each other.

> **Tasty Morsel (of information)**: If you choose to drink alcohol use moderation, and eat food while you are drinking. This can decrease the chances of having a low blood glucose, and it can slow the effects of the alcohol.

Excessive drinking can also contribute to high blood glucose, which can lead to problems over time. The biggest offender is the mixers. If you drink rum and Coke® or a Screwdriver, imagine how much carbohydrate is in the mixer (Coca Cola® or orange juice). Margarita mix is also very high in sugar. There are ways to deal with this: use Diet Coke®, diet tonic, or "lite" juices.

> **Tasty Morsel (of information)**: My recipe for Margaritas includes using lime juice ("lite," if possible) and sugar-free lemon-lime soda. This drastically reduces the amount of added sugar. Another idea is to mix up some sugar-free lemonade and use that as the "mix." We now have "lite" Margarita mix available as well.

Try checking your blood glucose before and after a mixed alcoholic beverage. Once you have a feel for how much one drink raises your blood glucose, you can plan for the next time by taking insulin, cutting back on the drink, or going for a walk. Just like everything else, alcohol can be consumed safely and enjoyably *in moderation*. On the other hand, if you have a problem with alcohol and you have diabetes, please see a professional to get help.

Dietary Recommendations

The United States Department of Agriculture (USDA) published Dietary Recommendations for Americans in 2010. You can read the full report at

http://www.cnpp.usda.gov/Publications/DietaryGuidelines/2010/ and here are their "key recommendations":

- Reduce daily sodium intake to less than 2,300 milligrams (mg) and further reduce intake to 1,500 mg among persons who are 51 and older and those of any age who are African American or have hypertension, diabetes, or chronic kidney disease. The 1,500 mg recommendation applies to about half of the U.S. population, including children, and the majority of adults.
- Consume less than 10 percent of calories from saturated fatty acids by replacing them with monounsaturated and polyunsaturated fatty acids.
- Consume less than 300 mg per day of dietary cholesterol.
- Keep trans-fatty acid consumption as low as possible, especially by limiting foods that contain synthetic sources of trans-fats, such as partially hydrogenated oils, and by limiting other solid fats.
- Reduce the intake of calories from solid fats and added sugars.

- Limit the consumption of foods that contain refined grains, especially refined grain foods that contain solid fats, added sugars, and sodium.
- If alcohol is consumed, consume it in moderation—up to one drink per day for women and two drinks per day for men—and only by adults of legal drinking age.

And here are some additional tips for healthy eating habits:

- When eating a food that is high in carbohydrate, consider cutting back on the carb, or combining it with a lean protein or healthy fat in order to decrease the blood glucose spike.
- Wash, peel and cut raw vegetables like carrots, broccoli, peppers, and celery sticks ahead of time. Put a bunch in a bag and keep in the refrigerator, so they are ready when you need a crunchy, low-calorie snack.
- Eat meals (and snacks) at the table. Avoid eating in front of the TV, computer, book, etc. This leads to mindless eating and you can lose track of how much you eat. Seriously, try it. Eating at the table can help you take your time, enjoy your food and digest it better. If you slow down when you eat, you may be less likely to shovel it down and be hungry for more a little while later.
- Serve your portion of a meal or snack onto a plate/bowl and put the package/container away. Eating out of a container (for example, chips, ice cream, crackers, bag of grapes, etc.) can lead to mindless eating and, again, you can lose track of how much you eat.
- Use a measuring cup to measure a serving the first few times you eat/drink something. Memorize where the serving amount falls in the glass or bowl, and after a while you can eyeball it and get

the right amount. This is especially helpful for foods that are hard to eyeball amounts, such as pasta, rice and corn. You may decide to use a measuring cup to serve them every time, and then you will know exactly how much you are getting. When you get really used to how much pasta is on your plate, you'll get better at estimating what you are getting in a restaurant.

- Prepare more meals at home than you eat out at a restaurant, convenience store or fast food establishment. Take your lunch – and snacks – to work.
- Eat snacks if they help you not to overeat at meals (or if you take a medication that requires a snack), but don't feel that you have to eat snacks because you have diabetes.
- Use a smaller plate!

> **Tasty Morsel (of information)**: Plate sizes have been increasing since the 1940s. The typical dinner plate is approximately 12 inches in diameter today, yet if we ate on 10-inch plates it is estimated that we'd decrease our calories at each meal by 22% (8)!

Special Note for Pregnant Women with Diabetes

Sometimes women with diabetes are still told they can't or shouldn't get pregnant. As you can imagine, women with diabetes *can* get pregnant, and as far as what they should or shouldn't do, well, that's up to them. If you've been told this, consider getting a second opinion, preferably from a health care professional who has experience with diabetes and pregnancy.

Pregnancy is hard without diabetes, and with diabetes it's even harder because it requires a lot of work. During pregnancy, women with diabetes not only have themselves to care for, but they also take precautions to keep their fetus (baby-to-be) safe and healthy. Managing diabetes during pregnancy is well worth the workload when a healthy mom delivers a healthy baby.

When I was pregnant, I found it easiest to avoid foods/beverages that drastically raised my blood glucose. For example, raw carrots made my blood glucose high when I was pregnant, even though this does not happen when I'm not pregnant. Cooked carrots are known for causing a blood glucose spike, but I don't eat cooked carrots, as a rule, so I didn't worry about that. You will quickly figure out which foods spike your blood glucose by checking your blood glucose frequently – which is what you do when you are pregnant. Juice is particularly notorious for quickly raising blood glucose. Some people choose to drink juice and/or regular (sugared) soda and compensate with exercise or medication. During pregnancy, however, it makes sense to avoid juice and regular soda so you don't risk spending time in the high blood glucose zone. Of course, if you are constantly sick or nauseated and juice/soda is the only way you can get your calories in, please discuss a plan with your health care provider.

Chapter 3
Three Squares a Day (or not)

When I eat breakfast, I can't stop eating all day long.
30-something female with type 1 diabetes

I have been known to say "I never miss a meal," and for the most part that's true. But it's not the case for everyone. Some people don't follow the typical breakfast-lunch-dinner routine that most of us think of when planning our meals. Some people skip meals, others have unusual or unpredictable schedules. For shift workers, "breakfast" may be eaten in the afternoon or evening. It is important to meet with your health care provider to figure out what works best for you and your blood glucose management, when it comes to meals. Let your health care provider know what your typical schedule and meals look like, and they can help you make any necessary adjustments, or at least provide suggestions. Although there may be a lot of pressure to eat three meals a day, the key to managing diabetes successfully and having healthy outcomes, is to do what works best for you and your body. In this chapter I will discuss the three meals that are typical in my approach to managing diabetes. Please take from it whatever helps or informs you, and leave what doesn't apply to your situation.

Breakfast

You might love it or hate it. Maybe breakfast "starts your day out right" or you feel obligated to force it down. Maybe you don't eat breakfast at all. For many, breakfast is the most controversial meal. Experts have been saying for a while now that breakfast is the most important meal of the day. You may have even heard or read that people who eat breakfast are more successful at losing weight. However, some people just aren't breakfast eaters.

For many (if not most) people with diabetes, the fasting blood glucose – first thing in the morning, before eating – is often the highest one of the day. This is due to the fact that two things happen overnight: first, in a fasting state (when you haven't eaten for several hours) the body thinks there is not enough glucose available, so the liver sends out stored glucose or produces new glucose; second, the body secretes growth hormone and cortisol in the wee hours of the morning. Both of these natural body responses cause the blood glucose level to rise, so by morning it can be elevated. The second one is often referred to as the "Dawn Phenomenon." A higher blood glucose level in the morning can be frustrating and challenging to manage. This first-thing-in-the-morning-higher-blood-glucose-level may also be a reason that some people don't eat breakfast.

It is true that breakfast is important because it provides the body with much-needed energy to wake up and start the day. People who don't eat breakfast may be likely to start snacking on less healthy foods by mid to late morning. People who don't eat breakfast may also overeat at lunch.

> **Tasty Morsel (of information):** Allowing more than five hours to pass between meals can lead to overeating at the next meal. Also, for some people, skipping meals can lead to health problems, especially if it causes people to overeat later in the day (9).

There are a few situations where breakfast is extra important. Metformin and Byetta are diabetes medications that need to be taken with food. The recommendation is to take metformin and Byetta with breakfast and dinner. Another medication that would require breakfast is a pre-mixed insulin taken in the morning. Pre-mixed insulins include 70/30, 50/50, Humalog 75/25 and Novolog 70/30. These are typically taken in the morning and evening. Because these types of insulin contain fast- or short-acting insulin, they must be followed with a meal in order to avoid hypoglycemia (low blood glucose). Chapter 7 has more information on diabetes medications and food.

So how can you incorporate breakfast without making yourself sick or late for work or emotionally upset? Start small. Eat a small amount of something you like. Many, if not most breakfast foods tend to be high in carbohydrate. People who follow a low carb lifestyle, however, find a variety of foods to choose from at breakfast.

> **Tasty Morsel (of information):** I can't emphasize enough that some people just don't eat breakfast. My son and I are breakfast people, and we have a hard time relating to my husband and daughter, who are not! It's important that we don't give people a hard time about breakfast. I compromise by giving my daughter a banana to eat on the school bus and she packs a healthy snack for mid-morning.

What about that quote at the beginning of the section? Do you find that when you eat breakfast you can't stop eating all day? Some people don't eat breakfast because of this problem. Some people find that eating a small amount of protein with breakfast fills them up a little more. Besides eggs, low-fat cottage cheese and yogurt are good options. You could put peanut or another nut butter on toast, English muffins, bagels, bananas or apples. At diabetes camp, we even put peanut butter on waffles and pancakes. As always, plant-based proteins or fats, such as avocados, are a good option.

If you just can't bring yourself to eat breakfast, for whatever reason, don't despair. Maybe you are a two-meal-a-day person. This can work too, especially if you space the meals somewhat evenly and eat consistent amounts. Perhaps a mid-morning snack and then lunch and dinner work better for you. The point is, as always, to make healthy choices: eat in a way that works for you and that you can stick with for the long haul. If you take metformin or Byetta and eat only two meals a day, take them with those evenly spaced meals. If you take pre-mixed insulin, ask your health care provider about other types of insulin that would work better with your eating schedule.

If you have a tendency to consistently eat less healthy items, you might consider substituting healthier foods in small increments. Maybe you could get to the point where you only eat pastries, etc., once a week. Then try once a month. Eventually you may find you eat those foods only occasionally, or that you don't even want them anymore. But if you still like a big, high-calorie breakfast, maybe the answer for you is to time your exercise for right after you eat in the morning.

When I asked my brother and sister – on separate occasions – what they remembered from when I was diagnosed, they *both* said, "no longer having sugar cereal in the house." I couldn't believe it! I have absolutely no recollection of there ever being sugar cereal in my parents' house when I was a kid. I have no regrets or hostility about not having eaten sugar cereal as a kid. In fact, I think it's just as well we didn't. Although it's all about choices, parents can encourage healthy choices by making them more readily available. The way I deal with this is to have healthier cereal options in the house every day. When we go on vacation, my kids get to choose their own box of cereal and it can be any kind they want. I've also heard of parents who let their kids choose the cereal, as long as sugar is at least the third (or lower) ingredient on the list.

Take a look at what you eat for breakfast. Sometimes we eat foods because we were raised on them. If that's the case, branch out! Granted, it's never easy to break out of a routine or habit, but you'll probably thank yourself in the long-run.

Lunch

Have you heard that lunch should be the biggest meal of the day? Years ago, people ate their largest meal at midday, and it was a hot meal to boot. That goes back to the days of farming and ranching, or at least having a job that allowed you to take enough time to sit down to a meal. Few people have that luxury today. Now most of us who eat lunch have something quick and often a "cold" meal like a sandwich. Some people eat leftovers, but let's face it, it's not a full-fledged meal when it's re-heated and shoveled down.

When you eat a large meal at lunchtime you have the rest of the day to work it off. Of course, with desk jobs and other sedentary lifestyles, the meal may not get "worked off." Many people use lunch as a time to cut back on calories. Some skip lunch altogether, others eat a yogurt or a salad and nothing else. However, it is just as important to get enough calories at a meal as it is to not overindulge. Not eating enough can lead to excess hunger, and therefore overeating, later in the day.

Once again, the important thing to remember is balance. Eat a healthy combination of carbohydrate, protein and fat. Don't forget fruits and vegetables. If you have a salad, you could sprinkle some berries or pineapple in it. Salad dressings are often a source of "hidden" calories. Try to stick with salad dressings that are made with olive oil, or other monounsaturated oils (see Chapter 2). Low-fat salad dressing may contain extra carbohydrate, so be sure to read the label. If you have a sandwich for lunch, try to choose a whole-grain bread. I aim for bread that has at least three grams of fiber per slice. You can find specialty breads that have even more fiber.

> **Tasty morsel (of information):** If a food serving contains five grams of fiber or more, you can subtract the fiber grams from the total carbohydrate grams. More recently, that rule has changed to subtracting half the fiber (if it's more than five grams). Either way, if you find food items with that much fiber in them, please let me know what they are! I have searched high and low for high-fiber bread. I was about to start making my own when I found one with four grams of fiber per slice, and I'm very happy with that.

Avocado is a healthy, plant-based fat that adds a great texture to a sandwich. Avocado can be an "acquired taste"; I started liking it at about age 40, so you never know. If you use lunch meat, be sure to buy as naturally-preserved meat as possible. Sodium is a concern with lunch meat. Although sodium does not affect the blood glucose level, it can contribute to high blood pressure, which tends to be a problem for many people with diabetes. You can also sneak some vegetables into your sandwich – cucumbers, tomatoes, lettuce, sprouts, peppers – just about anything adds crunch and/or flavor (and nutrients!) to a sandwich.

Soups are delicious and often comforting. Choose (or make) a soup that is full of vegetables for added nutritional value. Watch out for overdoing the carbs in a soup lunch: noodles/pasta, rice, barley, potatoes and corn are all carbs frequently found in soups. If you eat your soup with crackers or bread, the carb content adds up very quickly. You might try counting out one serving of crackers/bread and then putting the box/loaf away.

Tasty Morsel (of information): In 1990 the Nutrition Labeling and Education Act (NLEA) was passed. This act requires that all packaged food have a label that provides information about nutrients in the food item. In 2003 the Food and Drug Administration announced that it would start requiring information about trans-fats to be included in the nutrition label starting in 2006. On the nutrient fact label, remember to check the "servings per container" first, then look at total carbohydrates (grams per serving) and figure out how much/how many would equal 15 grams of carbohydrate.

Leftovers are great! Packing leftovers for lunch is a fast, easy way to prepare a meal. If you are preparing healthy meals at dinner/supper, your lunch will be healthy too. Use caution when packing leftovers, and pack a reasonable amount of each food item. It's easy to just throw in all of it, since it's in the container. Perhaps you can get two additional meals out of it.

Some people eat a little cup of yogurt and call that lunch. Again, not eating enough at lunch can lead to overeating at dinner/supper. Yogurt can be a good source of protein, and other nutrients; however, it may not be enough. If you are trying to eat fewer calories or healthier choices, add some fruit and vegetables to your yogurt lunch; maybe a salad.

Fast food is lunch for many people – even on a daily basis. You may be going out to a local fast food chain or eating in a cafeteria at your work facility, which may not serve the healthiest food choices. If you can, start packing your lunch at least part of the time. If this is not possible, try to choose healthier options at fast food places. Resources are available that provide the nutrition content of fast food. Ask at the counter for a printout of nutrition information for their menu items.

Whether you are looking for fast food or fancy dining, another helpful resource is www.healthydiningfinder.com. This website helps you find healthy food options wherever you are located. Try it out!

Dinner/Supper

Back in the day, when "dinner" took place at noon – a large, hot, sit-down meal – the lighter, evening meal was typically called "supper." Now it is not unusual for supper to be the largest meal of the day, and many people call it "dinner." It may, for some, be the only sit-down meal. What does a dinner/supper menu look like for you? Here is a breakdown of some typical items from the evening meal:

- Protein of some sort (roast, steak, chicken, pork, fish, beans)
- Salad or cooked vegetable

Steamed vegetables are healthier than microwaved or boiled vegetables, because they retain more of the vitamins and minerals. Fresh vegetables are always best, but if that's not an option then frozen is better than canned. This is because canned vegetables are typically packed in a lot of salt. Salads are great; watch out for high-calorie salad items such as croutons, cheese and high-calorie dressing. Olive oil-based salad dressings are the healthiest choice. Start with a salad, so you won't have room to overeat the rest of the meal. Pack lots of vegetables in your salad (not just lettuce): carrots, tomatoes, peppers, mushrooms, radishes. Vegetables are full of antioxidants, and we cannot get enough of them. One-half cup of cooked vegetables or one cup of raw vegetables equals a "serving." One vegetable serving has five grams of carbohydrate, which means that if you eat three servings, they will count as a carbohydrate serving (15 grams of carbohydrate). Don't let this stop you from eating vegetables, however. Also, keep in mind that a "vegetable" does not include potatoes or corn. These are starchy vegetables and they fall strictly in the carbohydrate category. For many people one serving of cooked peas or carrots is starchy enough to raise the blood glucose level as well. Again, you don't have to avoid these nutritious vegetables; just keep in mind the effect they will have on your blood glucose and plan accordingly.

> **Tasty Morsel (of information):** If you prepare cooked carrots or squash (butternut, acorn) with brown sugar, don't forget to consider how this added carbohydrate will affect your blood glucose. Options include using a non-nutritive sweetener version of "brown sugar," use less brown sugar than you ordinarily would, or take a walk after the meal.

- Starch of some sort (potato, dinner roll, rice, pasta, corn)

It's very easy for the carb content of a supper/dinner to creep up. For instance, if you are having spaghetti and you add Italian bread – that can be a lot of carb! If you just can't live without bread, try whole-grain Italian bread and stick with one piece. Another idea is to go with whole-grain bread sticks. If you are having a potato with dinner/supper, you can skip the dinner roll. When it's a rice or pasta night, serve brown rice or whole-grain pasta with a one-third cup measure so you know exactly how much you're getting (1/3 cup cooked pasta or rice = 15 grams of carb). It's easy to eat three or more carb servings in a typical meal. With rice and pasta the carb grams add up quickly, which is why blood glucose can be high later on (and weight gain can occur). Although most people consider corn a vegetable, in the diabetes world it is starch or carbohydrate. If you are serving corn with dinner/supper, add another vegetable or a salad and consider the corn your carb for the meal.

Tasty Morsel (of information): Exception to all the rules: Thanksgiving Dinner! Thanksgiving dinner is basically one big carb fest. Think about traditional Thanksgiving foods – stuffing (dressing), corn in some form or another (corn pudding is my favorite), potatoes, butternut squash loaded with brown sugar, noodles, assorted breads and/or rolls, cranberry sauce, pie. Am I forgetting anything? If the turkey doesn't make you sleepy, the carb overload certainly will! At any rate, we must celebrate from time to time, and Thanksgiving is a good reason to do so. Talk to your health care provider to determine whether you need to adjust your diabetes medications for holiday feasts. It is also very important and beneficial to take a long walk after a big meal.

- Casserole or combination food

I am a big fan of what I like to call "straight-forward food." By this I mean separate protein, carb and vegetable dishes where I know exactly what I'm getting. As a result, I do not often make casseroles. The challenge with casseroles (and I do enjoy them; I was brought up going to a lot of "potluck dinners" at church) is that it is hard, if not impossible, to figure out exactly what you're getting in terms of carb, protein, and fat when you eat a casserole. It is certainly possible to estimate, though, and if you really enjoy these foods there is no reason to ban them from the menu. With a little trial and error, you can figure out how much carbohydrate is in a serving of a casserole. If you take insulin you can then make appropriate adjustments, and if you don't take insulin, some exercise after supper/dinner is always helpful. Another downside to casseroles is that they tend to be high in fat. The typical casserole has a cream (or cream soup) base, a lot of cheese, etc. If you can lighten up the recipe somehow, you'll be better off. Perhaps you could use yogurt instead of sour cream; add fat-free milk to cream-based soups, decrease the amount of cheese or try a low-fat cheese.

- Dessert

I grew up in a family that always ate dessert after supper. My motto, as a result, is "always end on sweet," and that may not work for everyone. I find that if I have a little bit of dessert I am satisfied. A typical dessert at home is fruit in some form and a little bit of dark chocolate. I have trained myself to be finished eating after I have my dark chocolate. If I'm out I either skip dessert or share with someone else. Then I have some fruit and dark chocolate when I get home.

> **Tasty morsel (of information):** Dark chocolate is healthy! In moderation, of course. Dark chocolate (or chocolate that has been processed as little as possible) has an antioxidant effect. Dark chocolate can also help lower blood pressure and increase blood flow to the brain and heart. Stick with dark chocolate over milk or white chocolate and keep reading up on the best kinds to eat – more information is being published all the time.

As I just mentioned, fruit is often dessert for me, and there are many different ways to have fruit: fresh fruit cut up in a bowl with a dollop of canned whipped cream; canned fruit; a fruit smoothie; or simply a whole piece of fruit. One thing to watch out for if you're having canned fruit is the sugar content of the juice. I go for the "lite" canned fruit and then I drain off the juice. If the fruit is in "heavy" syrup, consider rinsing the fruit with water to remove the syrup, which is full of sugar. Even if the fruit is in "natural juice," it just decreases the amount of whole fruit you get, so you might be better off pouring the juice off and enjoying more fruit. As usual, fresh fruit is best, but in the off-season, canned and frozen fruit are great too. Frozen berries make a wonderful smoothie. Sugar-free Jell-O and pudding (made with fat-free milk) are nice, low-calorie dessert options. They are great with fruit mixed in as well.

It's very helpful to learn how much of a particular type of fruit is in one serving, especially if you take insulin. For instance, a small apple, half of a standard banana, 10 to 12 grapes (or fewer if they are huge), and one cup of cantaloupe are all equal to a fruit – or carb – serving. Again, lists of foods and their carbohydrate content are readily available in books and on the Internet; you might want to create your own list of the foods you tend to eat most frequently and the amount of carb they contain.

Snacks

What about snacks? There is a long-standing belief that people with diabetes have to eat snacks (I think this message is also circulating about people living in nursing homes, diabetes or not). For people who take insulin, this started back when we had only a few types of insulin and they worked in such a way that when the insulin's action was peaking there needed to be food on board, which was often between meals. This set-up required between-meal snacks. When I was in second grade – my first time back to school with diabetes – I had to eat my snack in the principal's office. Although I got used to it after a while, this was actually quite embarrassing for me, because every day the principal would ask, "What did you bring for me?" For people who don't take insulin, the snack idea may have come from the belief that six small meals a day is a healthier approach to eating. As always, different things work for different people.

For those who use it, we now have new and improved insulin and we aren't necessarily required to eat snacks. Not to mention that many people with diabetes may be trying to lose weight, and don't want to eat extra calories between meals. On the other hand, if you prefer eating smaller portions several times a day, there is nothing wrong with that approach. Once again, it's about choices, and you can choose what works best for you. Which approach helps you feel full and satisfied and less likely to overeat? For some people this is the six-small-meals/snacks-evenly-spaced-throughout-the-day approach, while for others it's the no-food-between-meals approach. Snacks, if you do choose to eat them, typically consist of a carbohydrate serving (15 grams of carb) and a healthy protein or healthy fat. It is ok to stick with just protein or fat if you are limiting carbs. Some examples are listed here:

- Nuts alone or with fruit (fresh or dried)
- Sugar-free pudding
- Fruit and nut butter
- Milk and plain cookies
- Low-fat cottage cheese and fruit
- String cheese
- Crunchy vegetables and nut butter
- Vegetables and a healthy dip
- Low-sodium vegetable juice and nuts
- Yogurt

Portion-control

I'm sure you've heard a lot of people talk about "portions" and eating smaller portions. How do we know how much is a reasonable portion? One way to figure this out is to meet with a registered dietitian, who can give you some guidelines for how much to eat in order to manage your blood glucose levels and achieve or maintain a healthy weight. There are also "rules of thumb" that you can learn. There is the "plate method," mentioned earlier, where you think of your plate as being divided in three parts: half your plate is filled with vegetables, one-quarter with whole grains and one-quarter with protein. Another guideline is to eat an amount of protein that is equal to the size of a deck of cards, or the palm of your hand. Visit http://www.webmd.com/diet/healthtool-portion-size-plate for some more helpful portion guidelines.

One thing that I do from time to time is to actually measure amounts of food. I pour my Cheerios® into a measuring cup and then pour them into a bowl. I then eyeball where the Cheerios® fall in the bowl, so that I don't need to use the measuring cup next time. Every once in a while I'll check to see if I'm experiencing "cereal creep" by pouring my cereal in the bowl and then putting it in the measuring cup. This helps me check to see if I'm still pouring the right amount. Another trick is that I use the same type of glass for milk: I originally measured eight ounces (one cup) of milk and poured it into the glass and now I know exactly how far to fill the glass. I use a different type of glass for orange juice to treat a low blood glucose. This way, I know that I am getting four ounces of juice and that I won't be over treating (see Chapter 8). When I make pasta or rice, I often serve it with a 1/3-cup measure so I know exactly how much carb I'm getting (because one-third of a cup of cooked pasta or cooked rice is one carbohydrate serving). Sometimes I use a one-cup measure to serve my pasta, and then I know that I'm getting three servings.

> **Tasty Morsel (of information):** Keep in mind that eating plans are not set in stone. The way you eat today could change completely tomorrow. It's important to try out different approaches and find what works best for you. And there are many options! The basic principles of eating that I share in this book are what

work for me - they have evolved over time and will continue to do so - and it's ok if you prefer something different. The important thing is that you don't find yourself stressing about food, that you enjoy eating, and that you are as healthy as possible.

Diet is a Four-Letter-Word (literally)

What images does the word "diet" bring up for you? Likely not happy ones! The authors of *Intuitive Eating* (Evelyn Tribole and Elyse Resch) discuss the "diet mentality" and the damage it can cause. Nutrition management of diabetes (a.k.a. eating when you have diabetes) is not a "diet," it's a lifestyle. I don't think the word "diet" was originally intended to have negative connotations. Over time, "diet" has come to represent a short-term activity, while lifestyle is life-long. How many people can survive on a "diet" for the rest of their lives? We all know how that works. I hear all the lines: "if it tastes good, spit it out," "if you like it, you can't have it," etc. I strongly disagree with that (negative) approach. With a little effort and practice, it is possible to find or prepare healthy foods that taste good.

For example, you can eat crunchy vegetables instead of chips. A healthy lunch could consist of half a sandwich on whole-grain bread (or lettuce or kale if you don't want the bread) with tomato and avocado. Crunch on some carrots, grape tomatoes, and snap peas or even dip them in a healthy salad dressing for extra flavor. Have a piece of fruit for dessert and you've got yourself an amazing and satisfying lunch! If you are one who does not care for vegetables, I really encourage you to keep trying. Try all different kinds, prepared in different ways. You never know when something will taste good. Maybe you'll find a new spice you like that makes vegetables taste really good! Keep trying – for your blood glucose, for your blood vessels, for your long-term health.

What about fad "diets"? When you think of a "fad," what do you think of? Bell-bottom jeans? Platform shoes? Poodle skirts? Asymmetrical haircuts? All of these "fads" have come and gone (and come again, in some cases, despite the fact that we wish they would stay gone). Fad "diets" are eating plans that come and go. For the most part, they are a "lose weight fast" program that may not work long-term.

Right up there with "What can I eat?" in the category of most popular questions asked by those with newly diagnosed diabetes is "What diet is best?" David Katz, a well-known physician who specializes in nutrition, weight management, and chronic disease prevention, summed it up this way: "The best diet is the one you're willing to do." Check out Dr. Katz's work at www.davidkatzmd.com.

Low Carb "Diet"

The most well-known low carb diets have helped people take weight off very quickly. One of the concerns with low carb "diets" is that people may replace healthy carbohydrate with unhealthy fats or too much protein. Another concern, which was mentioned earlier, is that as soon as people add carbs back into their daily meal plans, they tend to put the weight right back on and often put on additional weight (10). However, many people successfully manage their diabetes with low carb meal plans. If this works well for you, and you do not have a tendency to overeat carbs once you cut back for a while, talk to your health care provider about the best way to make this work. A good book that discusses the science behind a low carb lifestyle is *The Art and Science of Low Carbohydrate Living* by Jeff Volek and Stephen Phinney.

Mediterranean "Diet"

You have probably heard about the Mediterranean "diet," which is actually more of a lifestyle. This meal plan is based on the traditional eating habits of people who live in the countries that border the Mediterranean Sea. It is known for emphasizing fresh fruits and vegetables; beans and legumes; whole grains; nuts; fish, poultry and lean red meat; wine in moderation; and olives and olive oil. The Mediterranean "diet" also promotes moderation and healthy portion sizes, eating in the company of others, taking time to savor and enjoy food, and other healthy lifestyle habits. Since this pretty much sums up everything that is recommended for everyone, we may need to plan a trip to Greece or Italy to study this approach in more depth…

In case you weren't already convinced, the Mediterranean "diet" can reduce the risk of cardiovascular disease. People who consume a Mediterranean "diet" are likely to lose weight, lower body mass index, reduce blood glucose levels and reduce inflammation (this is what leads to heart disease). For people who have already had a heart attack, following the Mediterranean "diet" can help them prevent a second one.

Vegetarian "Diet"

People with diabetes can successfully obtain all the necessary nutrients from a vegetarian "diet." Vegetarians do not usually have a problem getting the protein they need; however, it's important to be conscious of getting protein from plant sources such as beans, nuts, nut butters, peas, and soy products. Vegetarians who eat dairy can get protein from milk products, and eggs are a good source of protein for those who include them in their meal plan. Vegetarians need to make sure they get enough vitamin B-12 by eating B-12 enriched foods or taking a B-12 supplement.

Glycemic Index

The glycemic index is a tool for figuring out how fast the carbohydrate foods you eat raise your blood glucose. The glycemic index

(GI) is a ranking of carbohydrates on a scale from 0 to 100 according to the extent to which they raise blood glucose levels after eating. Foods with a high GI are those which are rapidly digested and absorbed and can result in marked fluctuations in blood glucose levels. Low GI foods are more slowly digested and absorbed, produce more gradual rises in blood glucose and insulin levels, and have proven benefits for health. Low GI "diets" can improve both glucose and lipid levels in people with diabetes (type 1 and type 2). They have benefits for weight management because they help manage appetite and delay hunger. Low GI "diets" can also reduce insulin levels and insulin resistance.

Some healthy foods, such as carrots and beets, come out high on the glycemic index, which can cause people to mistakenly strike them from the meal plan. Many people find the glycemic index effective in helping them successfully manage their diabetes. For more information visit www.glycemicindex.com.

Between-meal Munchies and the Bewitching Hours

Are you challenged by feeling the need to snack or "graze" between meals? For me, the biggest challenge is right after work. I call this the "bewitching hour(s)." I try hard to eat something that won't make too much difference to my blood glucose before supper. Some days I'll have a handful of almonds or peanuts, and other days I will munch on some carrots and "dip." For a dip I like to use a healthy salad dressing like Newman's Own® Lite Honey Mustard. Any vinaigrette made with olive oil would be good too. I buy a huge bag of carrots, wash, peel, cut them up and store them in the refrigerator. This way, there's no work involved when I want an easy snack. You can also buy a bag of ready-to-serve, peeled mini-carrots. Another idea is a can of vegetable juice (low-sodium, of course). This can be a great pick-me-up when you just want to get by until the next meal. The trick here – if you haven't caught on already – is to have quick, healthy options available so that you don't even have to think about it. Once I get that snack in me, I'm good until supper. If the challenge is "grazing," you may choose to do a little more work with yourself. You can use distraction techniques – is there a project you want to work on? Make a list! Have a (healthy) snack after you have crossed three things off your list.

Some people choose to make food the enemy. They tend to think of diabetes as a war and food as a battle. This mentality can lead to a lot of anger and very negative feelings. This approach can stem from frustration or even fear. I choose to respect diabetes rather than fear it. I find that respect is a healthy, positive approach to this disease, and one that helps me stay focused and motivated. Fear can keep us from doing the things we need to do to take care of ourselves. In addition, fear, negative feelings, and anger can trigger the body's stress response which can raise the blood glucose further. That just defeats the whole purpose of managing diabetes.

It cannot be overstated that the most successful weight loss programs are often those that help people take off weight slowly, gradually, over time. No one got to their present weight overnight, and no one can safely and successfully lose it overnight. The goal is to successfully change your lifestyle – to change your daily eating and exercise (and stress management) habits – and keep the new ones for the rest of your life.

Change is hard. Change is frustrating. There are small successes and big failures along the way. If you stick with it, and don't beat yourself up when you slip or fall, you can do it. Once your new lifestyle becomes habit, you may even like it! You will most likely feel a lot better – have more energy, get more done, have more confidence and self-esteem. Once you do change your lifestyle and start feeling good physically, enjoying it and feeling great about yourself, it may become difficult to be around those people and places where unhealthy habits prevail. You will need to figure out a plan for how to handle this.

If a fad "diet" helps kick-start your weight loss program, then it's fine to use one. When it's time to reintroduce carbohydrates into your diet, be sure to eat healthy ones: fruits, vegetables, legumes, whole grains, and low-fat dairy. There is a lot more to read and learn about fiber, fats/oils and nutrition in general. You can find all sorts of information on the Internet. While there are many dependable websites, there are also some to avoid. Check with your health care provider if you have questions about what you learn on the Internet.

Special Note for Those Whose Meal Plan or Times are Different

If, for cultural, religious, or other reasons, you follow a meal plan that is different from what I've described so far, please know that you can still make healthy choices. Work with a dietitian or other health care provider to determine appropriate foods and amounts for your body's needs. *You do not have to give up everything you love*; you may just want to make some changes in how much you eat or how you combine different foods. If you have a different schedule, you can also work with a health care professional to figure out the best way to handle food and diabetes.

Chapter 4
Lemon Twist and the Art of Diabetes Management

Exercise cuts into my TV time
60-something male with type 2 diabetes

A special treat for my family was to drive over to a neighboring town and get a soft-serve ice cream cone on a Friday night after supper. There were a couple of places we liked. Both were drive-up ice cream bars where we would go up to the counter, order our ice cream and then stand around and eat it (basically in the parking lot). My mother came up with a brilliant idea: Lemon Twist after ice cream. The Lemon Twist was a rubber contraption that went around the ankle with a plastic lemon on the end (released in 1975 by Chemtoys – look it up, it'll bring back memories). The object was to spin the lemon around while jumping over it. I don't remember when or how the Lemon Twist arrived in our house, but I remember bringing it with us when we went for ice cream. I would eat my ice cream and then do 100 "lemon twists" in the parking lot. I have to hand it to my mom for coming up with that one – what a great idea! We didn't know about dosing extra insulin for extra food (see Chapter 7) in those days. I took the same dose of insulin every day (once a day) until I saw my "team" and they decided if changes were necessary.

> **Tasty Morsel (of information):** When I was a kid, I was told that I could choose between vanilla, chocolate, strawberry, or peach ice cream. I honestly have no idea where that thinking came from. We know that ½ cup of ice cream is approximately 1 carb serving and 2 fat servings. Perhaps the thinking was that with those basic flavors we could be sure of the "exchanges," whereas with flavors such as bubble gum, chocolate chip, etc. we

73

couldn't be sure. These days we have basic flavors and we have exotic flavors (I'm thinking of Milky Way and Snickers among others). There is regular fat ice cream and premium (higher fat) ice cream, such as Ben & Jerry's or Haagen Dazs®. You can do your own experimenting, but the important thing, as always, is moderation.

Another idea of my mother's was having me run around the (outside of the) house after eating a homemade cookie or brownie. I truly appreciate the fact that she did not restrict me from eating those things, but instead figured out a way to at least partially counteract the sugar I was consuming. Physical activity is a critical part of managing diabetes. After attitude, I think it's the most important part, and that may be a bold statement. However, if someone with diabetes is active, several things tend to happen: they tend to make healthier food choices without thinking about it (as much); they tend to be happier/more well-adjusted (manage stress); their bodies tend to work more efficiently; they tend to lose or maintain weight; they tend to sleep better; and they tend to feel stronger and have more energy. In addition, physical activity decreases the symptoms of depression.

There really is an art to diabetes management. For example, when I ask a patient, who takes insulin, how they dose their insulin for a certain situation, they respond, "I can't explain it. I just know." For all the science (and there's a lot) that goes into managing diabetes, there's a lot of art too! This can be especially true with exercise. For those of you reading this who have type 2 diabetes, the exercise message is pretty straight forward: *exercise lowers blood glucose*. I think of it as making the body work more efficiently. Since type 2 diabetes is basically a case of the body being inefficient (at using insulin and metabolizing glucose), wouldn't the first line of attack be something that improves this? Not only does physical activity lower blood glucose in the short-term, but since being active can help you lose weight and weight loss can lower blood glucose, exercise is truly the gift that keeps on giving. In addition, regular exercise increases muscle tone. Muscle tone is the activity going on in your muscles when you are *not* being active. So if you make exercise a regular part of your life, even when you are not engaging in physical activity, your body is still working, burning calories and overall performing more efficiently. Exercise is also important and beneficial for those with type 1 diabetes, it just gets a little more complicated, and we'll discuss this later in the chapter.

> **Tasty Morsel (of information):** It may appear that I use the terms physical activity and exercise interchangeably in this chapter. Physical activity and exercise are both movements of our bodies that we do voluntarily. The difference is that physical activity is any movement of your body, while exercise is a planned activity that is structured and repetitive, and one that increases your heart rate for a sustained period of time.

Exercise and Eating Habits

Many people find that when they exercise consistently, they do not crave unhealthy foods as much, if at all. Healthy habits beget healthy habits! Depending on what type and how much exercise someone is doing, they may actually require *more* calories, but these calories are being burned off. Because some people don't make changes to their eating habits – for whatever reason – exercising provides a buffer, of sorts. If you choose to eat donuts every Sunday, and you take a walk after you eat them, you are doing your body a big favor. While high-fat foods can raise triglyceride and LDL levels ("bad" cholesterol), exercise raises HDLs ("good" cholesterol), so exercise helps protect you from heart disease. Some research studies have shown that even if someone is overweight, being active makes them healthier than those who don't exercise (11). It is important to stay hydrated when you are exercising. Be sure to drink plenty of water throughout each day.

Exercise and Stress Management

Exercise helps our bodies produce endorphins, which are natural feel-good substances. Find a form of exercise that you enjoy and your endorphins will kick in (reality check: if you are doing something you hate or are in physical pain from it, your endorphins won't win). This helps take your mind off stressful events, come up with solutions to problems you are experiencing, clear your mind when it is "racing" with a million thoughts, or just take time to think about nothing! One catch, though, is that when you get to the point where your day is not complete without your exercise routine, you need a back-up plan for when plans change. For a long time I walked on Mondays, Wednesdays, Fridays and Saturdays. One Wednesday my husband had to be driven to surgery (the nerve!). I literally had to do some self-talking to stay calm and figure out when I could walk later in the day. It all worked out just fine – but my family knows, by the way, that I am a happier person when I have had my walk.

Get in the habit

When you are just starting out with exercise, it's easy to blow it off if the schedule changes or something comes up. Try hard to stick with it. Again, choose an activity that you enjoy and a time that works for you and keep at it until it's a habit. Start small, for instance, walk to the end of the block and back. I talk to many patients who cannot imagine fitting exercise into their busy schedule. What about someone who works nights, sleeps for a few hours during the day and then has kids to take care of as soon as they wake up? What about the person who works two or three jobs? I imagine that if your life looks something like that – you are stressed!! You would especially benefit from adding exercise to your day or week. Could you take a break at work and go for a walk? Could you stop and use a gym on your way home from work? Could you use a work-out tape with the kids in the house?

The man who said the quote at the beginning of the chapter had just had knee replacement surgery. He was responding to my suggestion that he continue exercising regularly after he completed physical therapy for his new knee. When he said that exercising would interfere with his TV-watching, we discussed getting a piece of indoor exercise equipment that he could place in front of his TV. I am very aware that this type of equipment is expensive, and not everyone can afford to buy it. This patient, however, informed me that used treadmills can be found for "pennies" all over the place! I'm not sure if this is always the case, but it's worth doing a little research – in the newspaper or online – to see if there is a piece of inexpensive exercise equipment for sale near you. And to repeat for emphasis, if you ever have to go through physical therapy for any reason, you can take advantage of being on a regular schedule of exercising and continue to do it afterward. If you find that you are more likely to actually do the exercise if you are accountable to someone, make appointments with a personal trainer or coach, or exercise with a friend (who won't let you off the hook). Some physical therapy facilities will allow you to use their equipment or at least suggest another facility if this is not an option.

I am not typically a group exerciser. I really enjoy walking, and most of the time I enjoy walking alone. This is my "Jane-time." I also enjoy going for walks with my kids, husband, a friend, etc., but I don't usually consider that my work-out. I have joined a gym at least three times in my life, and all three times I used the gym *maybe* three times. Now I know for sure that I do not need to join any more gyms. I also know that getting in my car and driving to an exercise place is not likely to happen (although I have started hiking lately, so you never know). As a result, I have two walking routines: one is my treadmill in my garage (works well with kids of all ages – strap them in for a video when they are babies), and I have an outside route that starts right out my door (when the weather is nicer). I also have an outdoor walking route at the places we travel to regularly. I am more creative when we are traveling somewhere new. More and more hotels have fitness rooms, and I try to use a treadmill when I travel.

If you don't like to walk, there are many other activities you can do: jump rope, lemon twist (although it doesn't look the same, and has a different name - "Skip-it"), swimming, exercise class, running, exercise equipment such as a stationary bike or elliptical or rowing machine. Think about what you liked to do as a kid and come up with some version of it now. How about a team sport? If you cannot get past your dislike for exercise, start by visualizing yourself exercising. Literally spend some time alone, thinking about what it would look like for you to exercise regularly – you never know what you'll come up with! If you are a very social person, enlist a friend or group of friends and exercise together. Start a snowshoe or kick-boxing club. If you find exercise incredibly boring, listen to music or a book on CD while you do it. You can download just about anything these days – including study materials if you're in school! If you physically cannot exercise, due to injury, weight, or something else, please consider meeting with your health care professional to find out what your options are. There are very few cases where exercise is ruled out completely. Finally, if there is any question about safety, talk with your health care provider about the best type and amount of exercise and *start slowly.*

I am living proof that it is possible to teach an old dog a new trick. Let this be an inspiration to those who don't care to think about, let alone participate in exercise. I started a group exercise class after spending at least twenty years saying that I'm not a group exerciser. What finally convinced me to give it a try was my discovery that despite increasing my walking to six days a week, I was not getting in better shape. I realized that science is right: if we want different results, we have to try different things. Although walking six days a week is good for stress management and gets my blood pumping, it just wasn't giving me the physical benefits I wanted. I started attending an exercise class that includes strength and cardio exercises in short bursts. I am using muscles I've never used before, and therefore, I'm getting a much more effective work-out.

Exercise and Health

When people with type 2 diabetes exercise, their blood glucose level typically comes down. I like to think of it as exercise making the heart pump harder, which makes the blood travel around the body faster and makes things work more efficiently. As part of this process, calories get burned because glucose is converted into energy by the body's cells. The food we eat turns into glucose, and what we don't use gets stored as fat. This is a very simple version of what goes on in the body, but let's just say that if we burn more calories through exercise, we store fewer calories as fat. This is why if calories in equal calories out, we stay at the same weight. If we burn more than we eat, we lose weight, and if we take in more than we work off, we gain weight.

People with type 2 diabetes who take medications, need to watch their glucose levels carefully while exercising. If numbers are consistently in the low normal or low range, a call to the health care provider and a medication dose decrease are in order. One of the main reasons to exercise is to maintain (or maybe even lose) weight, so if you are experiencing repeated hypoglycemia (low blood glucose), where you have to treat it with extra calories, you're defeating your purpose. Not all medications cause hypoglycemia, so check with your provider about that. In addition, it's important not to take more medication than your body needs, so if you can cut back on a dose or eliminate a medication because of your increased activity, that's a good thing!

People with type 1 diabetes have a few extra precautions to consider when exercising. Insulin's job is to lower blood glucose. If insulin is on board and working, typically the blood glucose level drops during exercise. Sometimes it drops too much and the person experiences a low. The best way to prevent hypoglycemia during exercise is to check blood glucose levels frequently (see Chapter 6), be aware of what's happening prior to exercising, and with experience, come up with a plan for food and insulin. I have found that I have the most success exercising in the morning after breakfast. I take my insulin, eat breakfast and then go for my walk/workout. I adjust my insulin dose according to my pre-breakfast blood glucose level and my planned exercise. I don't need as much insulin on my walk days as I do on my non-walk days. If my blood glucose is low before breakfast, I will not only take slightly less insulin, but I will also put some fruit on my cereal. Trust me; it has taken years of practice, trial and error to get this system down. And there are still days when it's not perfect.

Tasty Morsel (of information): Back when we had fewer choices of insulin, the types we did have worked differently than ones we have now. They also had very defined peak action times and long "tails" when they may still be working. In other words, they were less predictable. As a result, it was typical for blood glucose levels to run highest right after meals (for those on insulin). The recommendation, therefore, was to exercise immediately after meals (yes, even swimming). Once we started using rapid-acting insulin at mealtime (Humalog, Novolog and Apidra), things got a little complicated. Exercising first thing in the morning, before breakfast, can actually cause blood glucose to rise because of the dawn phenomenon (see Chapter 6). Once there's insulin – and food – working, exercise generally works better. Later in the day, however, can be a challenge because lunch or supper-time insulin might cause a low. It's very important to check blood glucose levels, make adjustments and work with a health care provider to figure this out. The process can be frustrating and take time, but you can and will get to the point where it all works nicely and exercise can become a regular part of your life.

For people with type 1 diabetes, there is a situation where exercise can cause blood glucose levels to rise and ketones (see Chapter 6) to form. This can happen if someone starts exercising with a blood glucose level that is too high. Unfortunately there is no good rule for what number is "too high." I was once taught that if your blood glucose is high because you ate more than you had planned, go ahead and exercise and it will most likely come down. If your blood glucose is high because you are sick, hold off on exercise – perhaps until you are no longer sick, but definitely until your blood glucose is in a safer range (check with your health care provider to see what he/she recommends). If your blood glucose is high for an unexplainable reason, consider drinking lots of fluids and taking a partial correction dose to get it down before starting exercise. You don't want to pull it all the way down to your target, though, as the exercise could then make you low. Again, your personal experience combined with guidance from your health care professional are the best ways to figure this stuff out.

Exercise and Weight Loss

I mentioned earlier that calories in and calories out determine how much we weigh (along with genes and other disease states). You can work with a dietitian to figure out how many calories your body needs to give you the energy to do what you need to do. When you add exercise to your routine, you may need to keep the calorie intake the same in order to lose weight. One pound of fat equals 3500 calories. That means that if you eat 3500 fewer calories each week, you will take off a pound of body weight. If you exercise enough to burn 3500 calories in a week, you will lose a pound - that would require a lot of exercise, though! It's probably more realistic for most people to eliminate 3500 calories per week by combining exercise with eating less food. Losing one pound per week is a safe and healthy way to take off weight. The more slowly you take it off, the more likely you are to keep it off for the long haul. As I mentioned earlier, regular exercise increases your resting muscle tone, which, in turn, helps you burn more calories. This happens because your muscles continue to work even after you are finished exercising, and because muscle tissue uses calories more than fat tissue.

If you are an instant gratification type of person, consider using some of the exercises in this book to work through your feelings about weight loss. Rally a support system around yourself (or be your own if you have to, or if that works better for you) and teach yourself to gradually make changes that will become part of your lifestyle. Adding exercise to your daily or weekly routine will pay off in big ways.

Exercise and Sleep

Anything you read will tell you that people who exercise regularly get better – and more! – sleep. They fall asleep faster and they stay asleep longer. This can decrease the need for prescription sleep medications, and can decrease daytime sleepiness (caused by the medications and/or the lack of sleep). People who get better sleep have an easier time getting up in the morning, getting through their day and being productive. Sleep is critical to long-term health (12). People who don't get enough sleep or good quality sleep, are at much higher risk for heart disease, cancer, obesity and diabetes. Poor quality and quantity of sleep also contribute to daytime irritability. I know it's true for my kids (of course, they hate when I say that). Not getting enough sleep may cause the release of stress hormones that can ultimately increase the rate of heart attack and stroke. Poor sleep can even contribute to elevated blood glucose – talk about fighting your efforts. Finally, there are a few people who can actually function and stay healthy with only a few hours of sleep each night. This is still not healthy for them in the long-run; we all need to take sleep very seriously.

> **Tasty Morsel (of information):** Sleep apnea is a breathing disorder that occurs during sleep. People who have sleep apnea actually stop breathing for a period of time, until they wake up and start breathing again. This pattern of breathing cessation, followed by disturbed sleep is a *major* risk factor for negative health outcomes, including heart disease. Unfortunately, people with type 2 diabetes very frequently also have sleep apnea. Snoring is one of the most obvious signs of sleep apnea, along with daytime sleepiness. If you snore and you have diabetes, it is in your best interest to get checked for sleep apnea. Ask your health care provider about having a sleep study.

Exercise and Strength/Energy

Without having a lecture on human physiology, let's just say that exercise literally helps our bodies make more energy. This happens especially with aerobic exercise, where we take in lots of oxygen. Oxygen (in addition to glucose) is the fuel our body's cells need to make energy the most efficient way. Aerobic exercise makes our hearts pump more efficiently, sending oxygenated blood around our bodies. Aerobic exercise consists of lower-intensity activities that are maintained for a longer period of time. Examples include walking, running, dancing, swimming, and bicycling.

Anaerobic exercise, or strength training, is good for us too. This type of exercise increases muscle mass and keeps our bodies lean. Anaerobic exercise produces energy without oxygen. Anaerobic activities are high-intensity and are performed in short bursts, such as weight lifting and sprint running. Our overall health and protection from disease improves when our bodies are in the efficient state resulting from a combination of aerobic and anaerobic exercise. Both types of exercise make us stronger. Bone health and strength are greatly improved with regular exercise, as well as heart health and muscle strength. In my experience, exercise also helps people think more clearly.

Exercise and Stretching

Just like people without diabetes, it's a good idea for those with diabetes to stretch routinely when they exercise. The purpose of stretching is to warm up the muscles and prevent injury. This is a very important part of being active, so that you can *stay* active. If you get a muscle injury you can't exercise until it heals. This can lead to getting out of the habit and having to start all over again. It's overwhelming and exhausting just thinking about that. Not to mention injuries hurt. If you have to seek medical attention, that costs money. There's just nothing good about getting injured, so please stretch! Strength exercises are also important, so that your muscles and joints will get and stay in shape. If you are not familiar with stretches and strength exercises, check out a book from your local library, or talk to an expert in the field (physical therapist, exercise physiologist, personal trainer, etc.). *Stretching* by Bob Anderson, is a good reference.

> **Tasty Morsel (of information):** Not only can people with diabetes exercise, but we can participate in extreme or competitive sports as well. There are many people who compete in all sorts of sporting events and have diabetes. There is even an organization for people with diabetes who are interested in exercise (Diabetes Exercise and Sports Association or DESA www.diabetes-exercise.org). For women with diabetes who want to challenge themselves, there is Team WILD (Women Inspiring Life with Diabetes). This group encourages women with diabetes to compete in sporting events: they work together and with the help of dietitians and trainers to reach peak performance. *Any* woman with diabetes is welcome to join them (visit their website at www.teamwild.org). Team Type 1 (www.teamtype1.org) and Team Type 2 (www.tudiabetes.org/group/TeamType2) are more competitive sports groups for men and women with diabetes.

Park Far and Walk

Throughout this chapter I have referred to both "physical activity" and "exercise." As a reminder, physical activity is any movement of your body, while exercise is planned activity that keeps your heart rate up for a period of time. Physical activity and exercise are good for us, and there are many ways to incorporate physical activity into your daily life, especially if you don't exercise regularly. I'm sure you can come up with even more.

- Park far away and walk (at the grocery store, mall, movie theater, etc.)
- Walk the dog
- Rake the lawn
- Use a push mower
- Play outside with the kids (baseball, Frisbee, fly kites, tag)
- Park farther and farther away and walk to work
- Ride your bike/walk to the corner store for supplies
- Take the stairs instead of the elevator
- Take the stairs instead of the escalator
- Walk the kids to the bus stop
- Do some gardening
- Vacuum/dust the house
- Dance
- Walk to the mailbox/post office
- Walk when playing golf
- Shop at the mall instead of online
- Get books at the library and wander the aisles
- Go window shopping
- Swim
- Go for a walk on the beach rather than just lying on a blanket
- Walk the perimeter of the field at your child's soccer game
- Walk your kids to school
- Walk around the zoo instead of taking the train or bus tour
- Putter

- Just move!

Watching television is relaxing, entertaining and brainless, and it has got to be one of the biggest things that keeps us from being active. Add snacking while watching and it's a sure path to disaster. If you are a self-proclaimed "couch potato," try making small changes toward a healthier, more active lifestyle.

- Put away the snacks – make TV time food-free so that you no longer associate watching TV with eating.
- Cut back on how much time you spend watching TV – decide which shows you can't live without and cut out the others. Replace them with another activity you enjoy.
- Spend the remaining TV time doing something active or even sort-of-active – put your exercise equipment in front of the TV and use it, or do exercises on the floor (leg lifts or arm curls) while you watch, or dust/iron while you watch.
- At the very least, hide the remote and force yourself to get up and change the channel!

Walk for a Good Cause

If it inspires you at all, consider the following exercise opportunities that actually benefit all people with diabetes: the Juvenile Diabetes Research Foundation (JDRF) and the American Diabetes Association (ADA) have annual walks to raise money for diabetes research. ADA also has a bike race fundraiser called "Tour de Cure" every year. These events take place all over the country, so check your local affiliate for the time and place and join them (www.jdrf.org and www.diabetes.org). Smaller, local diabetes organizations provide additional opportunities to exercise and raise money. Diabetes camps and

Lions Clubs (that regularly support diabetes camps) often hold golf tournaments and run/walks to raise money for programs for kids with diabetes and their families.

Never too Late to Exercise

I was once told that the exercise habits you start in college stay with you throughout your life. It was said in a way that made me believe I had to start then or I'd be doomed. Luckily I was in college at the time. I know now, however, that it is never too late to start exercising. And it is always too soon to stop. So regardless of how old you are, or what kind of shape you are in, or whether or not you went to college, you can still be active. If you have a physical condition that makes it hard to exercise, talk to your health care provider and find out what activity you can do to get your heart rate up. If you have arthritis, believe it or not, exercise can actually improve your symptoms (13). If you are currently exercising, don't stop! I am living proof that you can increase your exercise, start going to a class, get stronger, and even enjoy a workout.

A little exercise:

Write down barriers to exercising

_____

_____

_____

_____

_____

Write down what you can do to overcome these barriers

_____

_____

_____

_____

Write down ways you could exercise and enjoy yourself doing it

_____

_____

_____

_____

_____

Chapter 5
Help Yourself to Success

I'm afraid to eat.
30-something female with type 2 diabetes

Everyone is unique, including people with diabetes. No two people with diabetes are exactly alike, and there is no one way to manage diabetes. In fact, an individualized approach works best for most people. Figuring out what works for you is the hard part. In the following pages you'll find some suggestions based on what I tell patients and what patients tell me. You can experiment with as many as you want, but in the end only you can decide if any of these suggestions or something else works best for you in successfully managing your diabetes. Get in touch with yourself by really paying attention to your body. Figure out what works and what doesn't work. Here's an opportunity to do that:

A little exercise:

Make a list of what gives you energy

_____

_____

_____

_____

Make a list of what zaps your energy

_____

_____

_____

_____

Did food have a role in either of these lists? Have you tried many different "diets," "meal plans," "cleanses," or other approaches to managing your blood glucose and/or losing weight? Have they helped? Have they flopped? What is the one change you could successfully make and stick with that would help you improve your eating (and exercise) habits for life? What has to happen in your life in order for the change to take place? How can you make it happen?

Setting Goals

The first step is to decide how you define "successful management" of your diabetes. Make sure the goals you set for your diabetes management are *your* goals and not the goals of your health care providers or anyone else. For example, decide what blood glucose levels are your targets, according to where you are comfortable and what is realistic and safe. Your health care provider's job is to give you all the information you need to prepare for setting your goals. They can tell you, for instance, that a normal blood glucose (for someone who does not have diabetes) runs between 70 and 110 mg/dL. For a long time the generally accepted target blood glucose levels for people with diabetes (excluding pregnant women) were 90-130 mg/dL before meals, less than

180 mg/dL after meals, and 110-150 mg/dL before bed. Now we know that it works better when target blood glucose levels are set individually. Many people work hard to keep their blood glucose levels in a much tighter range than even these targets. Others use a more liberal target, and there is everything in between. You get to work with your health care professional to fine-tune your target to your own needs and decide what your personal goals are. Your provider can let you know what the research says. For instance, if you are completely new at this, or you are "checking in" after a long break, you may ask your provider, "What's a safe and healthy target for my blood glucose levels?" Your health care provider may then answer, "Research shows that if you keep your A1C (a measure of your three-month average glucose) as close to 6% as possible, your chances of having blood vessel damage and developing diabetes-related complications drop drastically" (14). You, then, get to decide what your goals are going to be. If you are ready to aim for a certain A1C, then your next step is to decide what you will do to achieve that. Your provider can help you set your goals by offering suggestions about changes that will make the most impact.

You also need to set your own nutrition, exercise and weight goals. Another goal may be frequency of blood glucose monitoring. It's a good idea to partner with your health care providers to gather information and come up with goals that are healthy and safe; however, you have to be invested in them in order to make them happen most of the time.

I frequently work with patients who say, "My goal is to lose weight," or "My goal is to have my A1C at 7%." I follow that with, "and what are you going to do to lose weight (or lower your A1C)?" That helps people get to a "measurable" goal – one where you can actually say

"I achieved my goal." For instance, "start exercising" is measurable; however, "walk for 30 minutes five times a week" is *easier* to measure and holds you more accountable. Another measurable goal is "check my blood glucose level twice a day, before and after different meals and write down the results." In Chapter 6 you'll have an opportunity to write down some goals. Are they measurable? Keep fine-tuning them until they are measurable.

All or Nothing Approach

Different approaches work for different people. This is true with diabetes as well as everything else in life. When we talk about food in particular, people with diabetes have different ways of dealing with it. For example, some people have an easier time eating in moderation than others. In an ideal world, everyone would have a "normal" or "healthy" relationship with food. We would all stop after two cookies, etc. But there is nothing ideal about having diabetes. So for some, moderation works, and for others, it's all or nothing. The "all or nothing" approach means these people have a tendency to overeat or not stop eating once they start (all), so instead they avoid certain foods altogether (nothing). This approach works very well for some people. For others the danger is that after a while they feel deprived or miss those certain food items, and they revert to old eating habits. This "failure" of sorts, can lead to feelings of self-defeat and further failure.

In 1991, I gave up chocolate. I had just spent four years in college, eating way more chocolate than I care to discuss. I never felt good after eating it, and I wanted to prove that I could live without it. I had a Junior Counselor my first year in college, who had given up chocolate for her New Year's resolution, and I was so impressed that I never forgot about it. The year after I graduated I decided to try it myself, so I gave up chocolate for a year, starting January 1, 1991. I found out that after avoiding chocolate for a year, I lost my taste for it. As a result, I continued to live chocolate-free for a total of fourteen years. At that point, I was pretty tired of eating around the chips in chocolate chip cookies, so I decided to eat them. One thing led to another and I began eating chocolate again. Interestingly enough, however, I no longer care for anything that is too intensely chocolate such as brownies or chocolate cake or chocolate mousse. And somewhere along the line I developed a taste for dark chocolate, which I had never liked before. I had always been a fan of less expensive milk chocolate candy bars (Reese's ® Peanut Butter Cups® being my number one source).

Although I know I have a tendency to be an "all or nothing" person - at least in some areas - I desperately want to find moderation easy. I have found that food items I have overdone at some point in my life, I now can eat in moderation or not at all. The two that come to mind are donuts and ice cream. I can take or leave either one of them, most likely because I overate them in the past. Take a look at the food items that cause trouble for you. Try to figure out why. Do you need to just stop eating them altogether or can you eat them in moderation? Some foods are a trigger for overeating. For me it's cookie dough. If I have a spoonful of cookie dough, it's all over. I'm better off not eating any (and I have learned, by the way, not to make cookies during PMS, if at all possible). A trick I have figured out after a lot of experience with this "vice," is to have only a spoonful of cookie dough after I've made all the cookies. In other words, I leave one glob of cookie dough in the bowl. Once I've eaten it I'm done and there's no more to tempt me.

I once had a conversation with a man who has chosen not to eat pancakes and syrup since being diagnosed with type 1 diabetes, and I respect his choice. For me, however, pancakes and syrup are an important part of life. I love pancakes and I typically have them for breakfast one day a week. I eat about the same number of pancakes, and I know how much insulin I need for them. I also exercise after my pancakes. I used sugar-free syrup for a long time; however, I currently use "lite" syrup. I like the taste better, I take insulin for it (because it still has quite a bit of sugar), and I find it easy to use just a little bit. If you like the taste of sugar-free syrup (which has definitely improved over the years), and if you are one to drench your pancakes in syrup, by all means, use it!

I hear some version of the quote at the beginning of the chapter *a lot*. People with diabetes are often afraid of food. This goes back to the messages that the general public has received about diabetes. People truly have the impression that they can't eat. Food is depicted as an evil villain that's going to kill them or get them in trouble. I once had a patient who came for an appointment after lunch. She reported that she had eaten Jell-O and nothing else. I struggle with finding an effective way to convince people that they can eat. They need to eat. It's all about making healthy choices, and we learn – through trial and error – which foods have the best effect on our blood glucose. The goal is to achieve the moderation approach in one way or another. The hope is that if we use moderation we never feel completely deprived of any one particular thing, so we don't overdo it. A negative approach can have the opposite effect. Thinking of food as the enemy can lead to stress and anger. If we are forcing ourselves to eat healthy foods and are stressed or angry about it, we have lost that balance. Although I do enjoy pancakes, I eat them in moderation. I don't eat them every day, and when I have them, I don't eat a lot. I also eat a lot of vegetables, so I have a nice balance in my overall eating plan - most of the time. There are definitely times when the balance is upset, and I choose more unhealthy foods. I don't beat myself up for these choices, however. Instead I acknowledge that it's not the way I want to eat long-term, and I get back on track as soon as possible.

Approaching food from a positive angle really helps. When I think of the overused word, "moderation," I really think of it as a healthy relationship with food and the thought processes that go into making food choices. If we focus on healthy choices and the good outcomes they deliver, rather than being afraid of food, we can enjoy food. Those who like a challenge can even work on discovering new, healthier versions of favorite meals. Once again, it's all about balance.

On the other hand, if there are certain foods (or drinks) that we simply have no control over, and need to omit them from our eating plan altogether, it is good to be aware of this. Eventually, if we stick to not consuming these items, we may not even want them. Giving up food is nothing like giving up cigarettes or alcohol. We have to eat to live. So to a certain degree, we have to figure out the moderation thing, because with diabetes, overeating even healthy foods like fruit or whole-grain bread leads to high blood glucose and eventually negative outcomes.

Planning Ahead

Planning ahead is an approach that helps many people with diabetes. Is it fun to plan ahead in terms of food? Absolutely not. Ok, not for me, but maybe for someone else it's a hoot. Planning ahead can, however, help you avoid overeating in certain situations. During a low blood glucose (hypoglycemia) event, for example, it is helpful to have healthy treatment options on hand. For instance, 1/8 cup of raisins, 4 to 6 oz. juice boxes and 3-4 glucose tablets (all equal to 15 grams carbohydrate) are healthy treatment options because in these amounts, they will bring your blood glucose level up about 50 mg/dL. When you are low it's hard to stop eating after only 15 grams of carbohydrate. For readers who have never experienced a low, you basically want to eat until the feeling goes away. By doing this, you can "over treat" and end up very high. This is just a vicious cycle, and a very common one.

Having treatment options with you means you never have to treat a low with whatever is available (junk food). Treating hypoglycemia with high-fat items such as candy bars, chips, or ice cream is not recommended for two reasons. First, these items contain a lot of fat and fat is broken down slowly, which means it will take a lot longer for them to raise your blood glucose. This, in turn, makes you more likely to overeat while you wait to feel better, and then end up with a high blood glucose level later on. The second reason not to treat lows with high-fat food is that they contain a lot of calories and will lead to weight gain. Weight gain promotes insulin resistance, which makes it much harder to manage your diabetes. I keep orange juice in the house just for treating low blood glucose. I only drink orange juice if I'm low – it's just one of those items that do not tempt me (maybe because I know how well it works at raising my blood glucose!). I use the same kind of glass and know exactly how much to pour to get my four ounces. It may sound crazy, but this is very helpful in avoiding over treating, since orange (or any fruit) juice is potent! There's more on treating hypoglycemia in Chapter 8.

As I mentioned earlier, planning ahead with healthy snacks and meals is another helpful idea. If you cut up raw vegetables and keep them in the refrigerator, they are an easy, virtually calorie-free snack when you need it and don't have time or feel like preparing. If those healthy snacks weren't ready to go, you might be more likely to grab something convenient that's less healthy. Planning your meals ahead can help you make healthier choices for meals as well. When you do your grocery shopping, get a week's worth of meal supplies, if possible. Include a vegetable, healthy carbohydrate, protein, fruit, etc. for each meal. This way, you won't have to go shopping the night of the meal (especially after work – yuck) and you will be more likely to eat a healthy meal than stop and get take-out. Plus, if you end up shopping at mealtime, you are much more likely to buy snacks and unhealthy choices just because you are hungry and want a quick fix. There is a list of healthy snack suggestions you can refer to in Chapter 3.

I once heard a great tip: buy fresh vegetables and leave enough time after shopping to wash, peel, cut them up and store them in the refrigerator right away. That way they are ready to go when you need a quick, healthy snack. I find carrots, celery, peppers, cucumbers and other raw vegetables much more appealing if I don't have to do the work right when I want to eat them.

Eating Outside of Your Comfort Zone

For some people it is easier to eat the same thing every day. I once met a woman who knew exactly how much insulin to take for each of the foods she ate. That is because she ate the same thing day in and day out. This may not be realistic for everyone, however. And certainly from time to time we have to handle food situations that are out of our norm. For some people, there is no norm. Experience and repetition play a big role in increasing our comfort level in different situations and with different foods. The ideal is to be able to manage well in any scenario.

From personal experience, I can tell you that the first step, when eating outside of your comfort zone, is to prepare mentally. You either know exactly what the scenario will be like (eating at your best friend's house or your relatives', etc.), or you have absolutely no idea. You can prepare by bringing your own food or calling ahead and asking what will be served. If you already have a good idea what will be served (in other words, it's always the same meal or type of meal), you know what you're in for. On the other hand, you may just have to punt. But you can still prepare mentally for having to punt: be flexible and open-minded. Think about what you will say if they are serving something you choose not to eat. Instead of saying, "I'm sorry, I can't eat that," which will just perpetuate the message that people with diabetes can't eat stuff, you could try something like, "I stay away from _____ because it makes my blood glucose wacky, but I love _____." You might even decide to eat something you ordinarily would not, just to be courteous, to try something new, or to avoid making someone feel bad (or to avoid the whole conversation about food).

At someone else's house...

See above. If it's a potluck, you can always bring something healthy. I often bring a veggie platter with a healthy dip, a salad with lots of vegetables and a healthy dressing, or a fruit salad. That way I know there is something I feel good about eating.

In a restaurant...

Restaurant eating can be challenging and frustrating. First, there are often huge portion sizes. If at all possible, share a meal with someone else. If that's not possible, eat half of your meal and take the other half home for the next day. There's nothing like leftovers for lunch – no fuss and they taste good! My husband doesn't eat fish and I like to order fish at restaurants, so sometimes we split a non-fish meal and other times I take advantage of being out and I order fish.

Next, there's the problem with food preparation. When you are in a restaurant, face it, you really don't know how the food is prepared. They could be adding extra carb or fat to your dish and you have no idea. The really expensive restaurants tend to prepare (somewhat) more healthy dishes and they also serve smaller portions – go figure! Watch out for meals with cream-based or sweet sauces. High carb foods will spike your blood glucose and high fat foods can contribute to keeping your blood glucose elevated for hours after the meal. When I eat in a restaurant, I always overestimate my insulin needs in anticipation of those unanticipated food extras. And I often have to take some more insulin once I get home.

A good trick to avoiding overeating in a restaurant is to order a salad. If you start with a salad it can begin to fill you up, so you don't have as much room for your meal. Then you can either split the meal or take some home and not be sad about it. Salad dressings can be more healthy and less healthy: olive oil-based vinaigrette vs. blue cheese - you do the math.

As far as dessert, you also have options. You can get a dessert for the whole group and just have a few bites. You can eat your own dessert and go for a walk after dinner. You can split dessert or skip it altogether. Sometimes instead of dessert I order a cup of decaf coffee and load it with cream and sweetener. It tastes like dessert and has slightly fewer calories.

On the road...

I have driven across the United States several times, and I can tell you that it is not easy in the eating department. Your options at most highway stops range from fast food to fast food. Oh, there are all sorts of varieties of fast food establishments, and many of them are trying to add healthier menu items, so they get a little credit. Also, in their defense, when you are driving cross-country you typically want to just get where you are going and not spend hours having meals. Every once in a while you might find a sit-down restaurant and want to spend the time. See above for suggestions.

If you are driving, however, you have another choice. You can pack a cooler for your cold foods and a box for non-perishable food. You have to get a new bag of ice every day or so, but you get to have the foods you know and love, it's fast, and relatively cheap – bonus! I have to admit that it took me years to start doing the pack-the-cooler-option (and I don't always do it on shorter road trips), but it is always well worth the effort. It's bad enough you have to sit in the car for hours on end, not moving, but then to eat heavy, high-calorie foods too can really zap your energy. And you need that energy for a rousing game of license plate bingo or silo/water tower-counting. Another suggestion is to do something active during rest stops. Bring along a jump rope or a lemon twist.

On vacation…

Picture yourself at an all-inclusive resort on a tropical island, or in a cabin at a ski resort, or a beach-front cottage. Whichever way you slice it, you come up with a lot of eating at restaurants (or bars). During your mental preparation work, you might need to prepare yourself for all that eating out. Think about what types of food you will or will not order (or how you will vary your choices). Will you start with a salad? What will you do about breakfast? If you have to eat breakfast in a restaurant several days in a row, you might want to make choices about which days you will have high-calorie breakfasts (pancakes, omelets, French toast, sausage and biscuits) and which days you'll opt for the lighter breakfast (toast, yogurt, or cereal and fresh fruit). If at all possible, consider staying in a condo or other place with a kitchen. That way you can at least prepare some meals on your own – save money and calories! And don't forget to go for walks. Invariably, you'll eat more on vacation than you typically do at home, so be sure to get some exercise and work it off.

Somebody reading this might be thinking, "If I'm on vacation, to heck with it, I'm going to eat whatever I darn well please!" This, of course, is one of your options. My only suggestion is that you might not feel your best if you eat a lot more food or higher-calorie foods than you are used to. You might have less energy for that golf game or other excursion than if you made healthier eating choices. You can weigh the options and make the best decision for you. If you take insulin and you decide to eat more, consider taking more background insulin (see Chapter 7). At any rate, you can always get back on track, so don't beat yourself up if you choose to indulge.

Camping…

I have fond memories of camping as a kid: my parents brought the cooler full of food; and cooked delicious meals over the Coleman® stove. I have great aspirations to do the same, but I have pretty much come to the conclusion that my camping days may be over. I never seem to have the energy to do the shopping, packing, food preparation, cooking and clean-up that would be required of my ideal camping trip. I won't get into my thoughts on not showering for days or sleeping on rocks.

If, however, you choose to go camping, you have the option to bring along healthy food choices. You can prepare meals over the stove (or campfire) and eat well in the great outdoors. And as an added bonus, food always seems to taste better when you eat it outside.

On a cruise…

As of the writing of this book, I have never been on a cruise. I have talked to several people who have been on cruises, though, and I have some definite preconceived notions regarding what it would be like. I think that's why I haven't gone. I picture one big buffet. I don't know about you, but buffets are a challenge for me. All that food, and I just can't let it go to waste. Plus it would be rude not to at least try everything, right? I know myself well enough to know that I would most likely overeat and then not have the motivation (read: vacation-mode) to walk as much as I would need to work it off. With that said, I do believe it's possible to eat well and exercise on a cruise. From what I hear there are all kinds of fresh fruits and vegetables/salads available. You can walk around the perimeter of the boat as much as you want (in addition to utilizing exercise equipment). So if you have serious will power – to eat healthy food and avoid the all-you-can-eat-24-hour-a-day ice cream bar and walk a lot – go on a cruise. Please let me know how it went; I'm going to go someday. Another idea is to take a friend who would make a pact with you to exercise every day. If you hold each other accountable, you can stick to it.

At college…

As I have mentioned in other parts of this book, I am not proud of the way I ate in college. I'm guessing many (if not most) people without diabetes would say the same thing. You've heard of the "freshman fifteen" (the weight people put on in the first year of college). This can happen when someone first moves away from home, regardless of whether or not they go to college. College is unique, however, in that it is *known* for leading to weight gain. The majority of college students eat in a cafeteria at least for the first year, if not all four. Cafeteria eating means freedom – all you can eat, and no parents breathing down your neck.

If you are about to head off to college, take some time to think about how you will handle food. I'm not suggesting that just thinking about it before you go will make it easy, but at least you can be somewhat prepared going in. Before I went to college, my mother told me that she had a student (my mother was a teacher) whose sister had type 1 diabetes. She ate candy bars all the way through college and then went blind. I think this was my mother's way of saying, "watch what you eat at college." Despite having these words in the back of my head, I definitely struggled with food in college. Food is central to all social events, from casual get-togethers to more formal school-sponsored activities. Alcohol is also prevalent in college. In Chapter 2 we discussed the importance of enjoying alcohol in moderation. People with diabetes have even more challenges (and risks) with alcohol consumption than those without diabetes, and college is not a time when moderation comes easily!

For some people, college is their first opportunity to truly exert their freedom and independence in terms of diabetes. If Mom and Dad had a watchful eye throughout high school, this might be someone's first real chance to eat whatever – and however much – they want. I went to a college where the majority of students lived on campus all four years, so we ate in a cafeteria. Despite the challenges of eating at a buffet every day, cafeterias do offer variety, and more and more are offering healthy choices. You can make a salad or find other vegetables, and plenty of fruit is available. You can also make other healthy choices such as fat-free milk and whole grains.

If you have access to a store and a refrigerator, you could stock up on healthy snacks (veggies, nuts, fruit) and bring your own supply to a social gathering. If you live off-campus you will most likely prepare your own meals. In that case, you are responsible for your own grocery shopping and cooking, so, as always, it's all about choices. This is the same for those who don't go to college, but leave home to work and live on their own. You might consider taking a nutrition class (any community college would offer one) or a cooking class or a community wellness or healthy eating class. In any of these places you can learn how to shop for and prepare healthy meals and snacks.

In the hospital...

Hospital food has never had a good reputation. I can still remember the food I was served in the hospital (in 1975). It actually wasn't horrible, but it had a certain smell to it. On occasion I will sense that smell and immediately I'm back in the "ward" (it really was a ward – a long row of beds in one room). Hospitals try harder now to have better food, but it is impossible for a hospital food service to know what or how much each patient eats at home. In order to provide the closest alternative, many hospitals provide menus that the patients fill out, which means you have some say in what comes on your tray. Many times that doesn't happen for one reason or another. Perhaps you arrived in the middle of the night so you get a random breakfast tray in the morning. If you are admitted for surgery, you will most likely have at least one meal before you are able to fill out a menu. I'm not sure if any hospitals have figured out a way to have patients complete their menu before they are admitted (for elective surgery, anyway). Great idea, but maybe not the first priority.

It is likely that you do have some choice in the hospital, so if you get a tray full of food that you would not eat at home, ask for something else. At the very least, you do not have to eat everything on your tray. I often hear complaints from patients about having too much food or too much carb on their tray. One patient said she ordered the chicken without the pasta, but the pasta came anyway so she ate it. If you get too much food on your tray, just eat the amount or choices you would eat at home and leave the rest. If it's too hard for you to leave food uneaten (maybe you were raised not to waste food), ask someone to take the tray away as soon as you are finished. Or put your napkin over the plate. Sounds crazy, but out of sight, out of mind. If you have to be in a hospital for an extended period of time, ask to meet with a dietitian to discuss your food choices. Open communication is the best way to get your needs met.

> **Tasty Morsel (of information):** When someone is in the hospital and needs a "clear liquid diet," they will receive a tray that contains caloric food items: regular (not sugar-free) Jell-O, regular (not sugar-free) popsicles, broth, cranberry juice, etc. The reason for the sugared items is that your body needs calories in order to heal and fight infection. As a result of getting caloric clear liquids you will still need insulin if you usually take it, and you might need insulin if you don't usually take it.

At a party (heavy appetizers)…

Let's say you're invited to go to a party right at the dinner hour. The invitation says "heavy appetizers." My husband knows how much I loathe this situation, because I complain every time. Heavy appetizers and I are not a good combination. I invariably overeat, yet don't feel I had a good dinner, so I eat more when I get home. Then I feel gross, have high blood glucose levels all night, and have to chase blood glucose with insulin. What to do? Of course, the first choice is to decline the invitation, but what's fun about that? You could just go for a little while, socialize, but skip the food and then go out for a real dinner. If it's potluck, I always go back to bringing something healthy. That way I know I can at least chomp on veggies all night if I have to. Another idea, if you are like me and still want something to eat afterward, is to make a salad when you get home. Salads are healthy and filling and aren't likely to do a number on the blood glucose. By the way, I finally figured out why I respond this way to "heavy appetizers." It's because with a meal there's a start and finish. With "heavy apps" you're never really sure what the entrée is, so you try everything and there's no definitive stopping point.

PMS (Pre-Menstrual Syndrome)...

Sorry, guys. I have to write about it, and you can skip this section if you want. PMS occurs during the period of time (days or even weeks) leading up to menstruation, when hormones are out of whack and a woman may not feel like herself. PMS does not affect every woman the same, and many girls and women do not have problems with PMS. For women who have had babies, PMS may change, get better, or get worse. Some challenges include food cravings (what I call "hormonal eating"), mood swings, irritability, angry outbursts, acne, depression, tearfulness, overeating, bloating, headaches, difficulty handling stressful situations or even situations that may not seem stressful to someone else. Because food can be comforting and because cravings can be common during PMS, there can be a tendency to eat more.

Some women experience higher blood glucose levels during PMS, so overeating makes them even higher. High blood glucose, in turn, can cause mood swings, lethargy, etc., so the problem is just compounded. For some women symptoms of PMS coupled with high blood glucose can lead to decreased motivation to manage diabetes and this turns into a vicious cycle. PMS, therefore, is something that women with diabetes really have to address. We can journal, exercise more, get massages or acupuncture, take antidepressants (talk to your health care provider if you think you would benefit from taking antidepressants during PMS), talk to someone, or try something else to manage our emotions and eating habits during this time each month.

Trick-or-Treating (Halloween)…

There are plenty of lists available that provide the carbohydrate content for a variety of candies. The thing to remember about trick-or-treating is that, typically, it is an athletic event. You walk around for up to several hours, knocking on doors, running away from scary people, and so on. I remember one Halloween when I was out trick-or-treating with friends. I really wanted to have a candy bar, and I hadn't touched anything in my bag when suddenly I realized that I had been walking for miles. Not only did I eat some candy, but it probably kept my blood glucose from going low that night. I recently heard about an adolescent boy who had a severe low (see Chapter 8) the morning after Halloween. This may sound surprising, but what likely happened is that he took extra insulin in order to eat candy the night before. However, because he and his friends had been running around the neighborhood and staying up late, he burned all those calories. No wonder he was low the next morning! This situation actually called for a little less insulin or a little more candy than usual. Frequent blood glucose monitoring (or continuous glucose monitoring) is the only way to stay in tune with what is going on.

Holidays in general...

Holidays are often focused on food, and holidays are a time when we tend to eat foods we don't eat the rest of the year. There are lots of great suggestions for getting through holidays without eating yourself into oblivion. Here are a few:

- Be realistic about your expectations of yourself – rather than planning to lose weight during the holidays, aim for maintaining your weight.
- Enjoy the company of family and friends, rather than focusing on food.
- Bring a healthy dish to a holiday gathering.
- Manage your stress level by getting enough sleep, exercising, and eating healthy foods whenever possible.
- Whenever possible, eat consistent amounts at consistent times – avoid skipping meals, as this can lead to overeating later on.
- Start your meal with a salad.
- Eat a salad or veggies before going to a party.
- Suggest that family and friends go for a walk with you after a meal.
- Drink plenty of water.
- Eat food slowly and savor it.

A little exercise:

What are some food situations that make you vulnerable to overeating?

_____

_____

_____

_____

What *do* you have control over when you are in these situations?

_____

_____

_____

_____

What works best for you?

To reiterate, for some people it is not only possible, but preferable to eat the same thing at the same times every day. Granted, this makes blood glucose management a lot easier. But many people want variety – they get tired and bored of the same foods day in and day out. And let's face it, eating at the same time every day is not always possible, no matter how hard we try. Why is it that meetings, practices, school concerts, etc., are invariably scheduled during the dinner hour?

It would be a lot easier to manage diabetes if meals were eaten at the same times every day. Because life often doesn't work that way, we are left to figure out how to make it work. What works for me is usually eating the same thing for breakfast, depending on the day. Most days I eat Cheerios® and fat-free milk. If I'm low, or if it's a walk day, I'll put fruit on my Cheerios®. As I've mentioned, I have pancakes once a week and one other day I typically have a fried egg and English muffin. This is my breakfast routine when I'm at home. If I'm away, who knows? This little routine works for me because it's easy and it gives me variety (in a routine way). Lunches and suppers are less routine, but I try to eat about the same amount of carbs and protein. I always eat a fruit and vegetable(s) at lunch and supper. I find this approach helps keep my blood glucose level more predictable; however, I realize that many people choose not to be so scheduled. Perhaps a more flexible schedule works better; it is possible to find a happy medium between routine and flexibility.

If you don't get tired of eating the same foods all the time, and you have the amounts figured out so your blood glucose stays where you want it – keep doing what works. If you need more variety in your life, that's ok too. With time, experience and being open to change, we can find ways to successfully manage food and blood glucose levels.

I grew up using the American Diabetes Association's "Exchange System" as a way of measuring types and amounts of foods. In retrospect I feel that this was a very effective and helpful system, and I had a very easy time transitioning into "carb counting" as a result. If you can get your hands on an ADA Exchange Lists for Diabetes book, it's a good resource for learning types and amounts of foods. The most current version is called *Choose Your Foods: Exchange Lists for Diabetes*. I recognize that many people find the Exchange System complicated, too specific, and constricting. Many people have bad memories of being on "exchanges" because they were told when and what they "could" eat. The problem was actually the type of insulin we had back then. Those "old-fashioned" insulins had very specific peak action times and they kept working for a certain amount of time, so food had to be on board at specific times. Luckily we now have much better insulin to choose from (and more coming all the time). Regardless of whether or not you take insulin, what we learned from the Exchange System was that eating a variety of foods is healthy. I think of it as a wonderful foundation for every meal that keeps me from simply focusing on carbs.

The media is full of information on food, some of it accurate and much of it not. More and more often we hear that specific food or food groups are "bad" or "good." As a result, people sometimes follow "diets" that cut back drastically or even eliminate certain nutrients. On the other hand, a simple approach to eating – one that includes a variety of foods in moderation – is probably best for most people. Again, find what works for you, talk with your health care provider, and make sure it's a healthy balance of the nutrients your body needs. If you are afraid of food, or if food is making you miserable, it may be time to rethink your approach to eating.

Control

People often say, "diabetes control" or "controlling diabetes." Do you feel as if you are in control? If not, why not? What parts of your life are out of control? What are some things (anything) that you do or could control in your life *right now*? Many of us eat when we feel out of control, and yet eating can lead to feeling out of control. This may be the case because of those situations that make us feel vulnerable mentioned earlier, or it may be caused by other stresses or pressures (work, relationships, etc.). Preparing for those situations can help increase the feeling of control. On the other hand, we can do something positive. Sometimes when I'm feeling out of control I *clean*. It may be the clutter or dirty bathroom that makes me feel out of control, so cleaning helps. Other times it's unrelated, but at least I can control how clean my house, office, or bathroom is. Besides, cleaning has extra benefits: it lowers blood glucose (it's active), has a great result/reward (a clean space – you may even find some long-lost treasures) and makes me feel good. Eating to gain control does none of those things; in fact, it makes me feel even less in control.

A little exercise:

Make a list of what makes you feel out of control:

_____

_____

_____

_____

_____

Make a list of what helps you regain control (or at least feel better when you're feeling out of control):

_____

_____

_____

_____

_____

Chapter 6

They're Just Numbers

Diabetes: the thinking person's disease
-on a diabetes camp t-shirt

When I was diagnosed with type 1 diabetes in 1975, we were checking urine for glucose. We did this by peeing in a cup, then putting five drops of urine plus ten drops of water in a test tube along with a "Clinitest®" tablet. This tablet reacted with the urine: it bubbled, got very hot and then turned a color based on the level of glucose. We used a color chart to determine how much glucose was in the urine. Dark blue was "negative," bluish green was "trace," and then we headed into the yellows and oranges. Dark orange was "4+," which indicated a lot of glucose in the urine. Aside from the obvious – it's pee! – the problem with monitoring urine glucose was that it was not a current measurement. Urine can sit in the bladder for hours, so there is no way to know what time period the reading represents. To make matters worse, glucose doesn't show up in the urine until the blood glucose level is 180 mg/dL.

In 1985 a nurse came to my parents' house and introduced me to blood glucose monitoring. I have no idea who sent her. I remember sitting at the kitchen table and learning how to use a blood glucose meter. It was called an Accu-chek®, and it was not the first meter to hit the market, but not too far behind. I had to put a ridiculously huge drop of blood on a "Chemstrip®," wait 60 seconds, and then wipe the blood off and put the strip in the meter. After another minute the meter gave a reading. Can you imagine having to take more than two minutes every time you check your blood glucose? Fortunately, over the years the amount of time involved with blood glucose monitoring has decreased. When I was pregnant my meter took 45 seconds. I actually had the timing down, so I could put the drop of blood on the strip, go to the bathroom and be back for the result. Now it takes about 20 seconds for the entire process from start to finish.

> **Tasty Morsel (of information):** The very first blood glucose meter was called the Ames Reflectance Meter. You can find an interesting history of blood glucose meters and home blood glucose monitoring by visiting www.mendosa.com/history.htm.

Back in the 80s, home blood glucose monitoring was a break-through. For the first time we could see what was going on right at the moment, instead of always being hours behind (as I mentioned earlier, urine can sit in the bladder for hours, so there's no telling how old the result is). Over the years, blood glucose meters have been improved continuously: they are smaller, faster, and take a fraction of the amount of blood that was required back then. Blood glucose monitoring is a valuable tool that allows us to see what's going on with our daily diabetes management. Checking blood glucose levels is an important part of diabetes management, because without it we are in the dark. The purpose of blood glucose monitoring is to provide information that the person with diabetes can act on. Knowing one's blood glucose level allows a person with diabetes to make decisions. The information we gain from checking our blood glucose level gives reinforcement when something is working or a chance to make a change when something is not working.

Just in case you are not convinced about how far we've come in blood glucose monitoring, here is a list of advantages of the meters that are available today:

- Downloadable (you can get software from the meter company – check their website – and download your readings into fancy charts, tables, and graphs)
- Alternative sites (you can obtain blood from a site other than your fingertips)
- Compact (no comparison to the huge boxes we used to have)
- Event "flagging" (you can mark readings as "before meal," "after meal," "exercise," etc., for easier tracking and averaging later)
- Capillary action strips (no more large, hanging drop of blood required – these strips actually draw the {very small drop of} blood right in so you can't miss)
- Blood ketone meter (there is actually a meter that measures blood ketones, so you don't have to pee on a strip)
- Large display (easy to see/read)
- Talking meters (great for the visually impaired)
- Backlight (makes checking in a movie theater oh-so-convenient)
- No code (more and more meters do not require a code)
- Updated lancing devices (easier to use, less pain)
- Meters with built in USB connection
- Meters that connect to smart phones
- Probably more since this book went to publication.

Some people have jumped on the technology bandwagon and really like to download their blood glucose results. Some use blood glucose apps on their Smartphones. They can create logs or even fancy charts and graphs to display what's happening at different times of the day. It's helpful to take the printouts to health care provider visits and make informed decisions based on the data. Some clinics have the software to download meters, so always bring your meter with you to your appointments. If you are downloading your meter either at home or at the provider's office, it makes a lot of sense to have all your readings on one meter. Some people like to keep one meter at home, one in the car, one at work, and so on. The downside to having multiple meters is that multiple printouts are hard to use for finding patterns and making decisions. If using multiple meters is the only way you will check your blood glucose, however, keep doing what works for you! And new apps are being developed all the time - watch for those that allow multiple meters to be uploaded into one database. Then again, if you don't care to use all the bells and whistles, you can always log your blood glucose readings on paper (or in a log book), and bring that with you to appointments. The most important thing is that you have your numbers available so you and your health care providers can look for patterns and make decisions about medications, food and exercise.

The meters we have now require so little blood that it is possible to use sites other than the fingertips to obtain the blood. Alternative sites include the meaty part of the palm of the hand, the forearm, the thigh, or even the earlobe. When I was a (diabetes) camper back in the 70s, we stood in line once during the two-week session and had our earlobes pricked for a "blood test." I don't remember ever seeing the results of the "blood test," but I do remember standing in line and getting poked. They said we don't feel pain in our earlobes. Hmmm. At any rate, I don't recommend alternative sites because, believe it or not, the blood in our fingertips gives a more "current" reading. If your blood glucose level is rapidly rising or falling, it is important to use your fingertips. This is potentially any time for people with type 1 diabetes. If someone specifically asks about alternative sites, I have no problem explaining how and where it's done (talk to your diabetes professional if you want to learn more about this). I find, however, that when taught how to poke the fingertips, people say that it does not hurt nearly as much as they had anticipated (if at all). The fact that we need so little blood means we don't have to poke as hard, so it hurts less. Plus the lancets we have today are much thinner than the old ones. A trick of the trade: poke the sides of the fingertips (some people have a little dimple there), not the very tips or the pads. The tips and pads are where your nerve endings are located, so you feel it more.

As far as lancing devices (more commonly known as the "poker thing"), trust me, they have come a long way. There used to be only one, and I called it the "guillotine." This dark blue, round, plastic device held one of those old-fashioned, blue lancets in full view. You would "cock" it back and then push the button to let it come crashing down on your finger. It had a horrible, loud sound and it pierced practically all the way through the finger (ok, I'm exaggerating, but that's the way it felt). I never owned one of these things. I preferred to just uncap a lancet and poke sans device. I even convinced my obstetrician's office to get a different lancing device because they had a "guillotine" and when I was pregnant I was in there constantly getting poked (or executed, as the case may be). Now that lancing devices are much nicer, I use one every day. The problem with using a lancing device is remembering to change the lancet. Although the official recommendation is to change your lancet every time you poke, many people reuse lancets, often several times. Make sure that you are the only person using your lancet, and keep your hands clean and dry before poking. If you are digging in the dirt or otherwise have dirty hands, it's a good idea to clean your fingertip extra well. It might be smart to carry alcohol swabs or hand sanitizer for times when soap and water are not available. Lancets will get duller each time you use them, so you might want to at least change it when it hurts or you can no longer draw blood.

Lancing devices have a "dial-a-depth" feature, so you can choose how deep to poke your finger. I recommend starting with it in the middle: if you don't bleed, dial up; if you hemorrhage, dial down. Finally, be sure to rotate fingers to avoid getting calluses or weird-looking, poked-up fingers. I poke my fingers between 4 and 12 times a day, but because I rotate them it's hard to tell that I poke them at all. And I can't emphasize enough: be sure that your fingers are clean and dry when you poke. Again, you don't have to use alcohol to clean your fingers (unless they are really dirty for whatever reason); water and soap does the job. If you have something on your fingers (cream, jelly, juice, etc.), it could alter the reading. This is why it is so important to wash and dry your hands before poking. If you do choose to use alcohol to clean your fingers, be sure it's dry before poking, because wet alcohol can give you a false reading.

Some meters require a code and others do not. If you have a "codeless" meter, you don't have to worry about it. Some meters use strips that all have the same code; once you enter the code the first time, you never have to worry about it again. Other meters require that you set the code with each new bottle of strips. Some meters come with a "code chip" that has to be inserted into the meter, while for others you must enter the code by pushing buttons on the meter. Please talk to your diabetes professional and/or read the instructions carefully so you know if your meter requires a code. Having the correct code programmed into the meter actually does affect the accuracy of the readings. If you have an older model of meter, and you can still find the strips that go with it, it's fine to keep using it.

One last thing about meters: every meter has a toll-free number on the back. If you forget everything you were taught about how to use your meter (you won't be the first), or if you are having problems with the meter or strips, call that number. The customer service people on the other end will help you trouble shoot the problem or even send you a new meter, if necessary. They are available around the clock, so do not hesitate to call if you need help.

> **Tasty Morsel (of information):** Many diabetes educators have blood glucose meters to give away, or you can always purchase one at a pharmacy. The cost of blood glucose monitoring is in the strips. It is important to find out which meter your insurance plan wants you to use, so it will cover the cost at the best rate; you will need a prescription for the strips. If you do not have insurance coverage for strips, you might consider a "generic" meter from a major pharmacy. The strips are often much cheaper. Talk to your diabetes educator for more information on which meter will work best for you.

Those of us who live with a chronic condition day in and day out, have a tendency to get in a "rut." We get so used to doing things the way we do them that we often don't consider other options. I have worked with many people like this and I am guilty of it too! Here are some examples: 1) I gave my injections slowly for years. I would put the needle right up to my skin and slowly push it in. I had been told that faster hurts less, but I just didn't feel like trying. Until I was pregnant and giving myself several injections every day. One time I tried giving it fast and I felt nothing! I've been injecting fast ever since. 2) Syringes and vials have never been a problem for me, so I never bothered trying an insulin pen. As a result, I didn't recommend them to patients. One day I realized this mistake and started recommending or at least letting patients know that pens are an option. And many, if not most, patients really prefer insulin pens. 3) I used the same brand of blood glucose meter for about 15 years. One day – literally – my health insurance carrier stopped paying for that brand of strips and I had to switch to a different meter (if I wanted the best price for strips). You would have thought I was a toddler if you had witnessed the tantrum I threw over having to change meters. Frugality won, however: I started using the "new" meter, and I survived the trauma and became adjusted to it. As much as I appreciate people's preferences and wanting to do "what we're used to," it's also important to try new things. Change can be good – you never know when you'll find something that will be a very good change and improve your diabetes experience.

Diabetes requires a lot of responsibility. While all people (with or without diabetes) are in charge of their own health, people with diabetes are also in charge of this chronic disease that must be dealt with on a daily basis. People with diabetes are often part of a larger "health care team," which may consist of a physician, nurse, dietitian, social worker/mental health professional, exercise physiologist, pharmacist, other diabetes educator, etc. Books, pamphlets and various reading materials often state something to the effect that, "people with diabetes are the central person in their health care team. They are responsible for

95% of their diabetes management." This is simply not true. *People with diabetes are responsible for/in charge of 100% of their diabetes management.*

Not one of those other members of the health care team is going to accompany us home. No physician, diabetes educator or other health professional is going to hold our hand while we sit down to a meal or watch us take diabetes medications. And they are certainly not going to make sure we exercise regularly by going to the gym with us. These are tasks that people with diabetes are responsible for doing on their own – 100% of the time. The choice to monitor our blood glucose is ours and ours alone. The information that we gather from checking blood glucose levels helps us make decisions for ourselves. Health care professionals can provide information, make recommendations, guide decisions, answer questions and generally serve as a resource and support; however, the individual with diabetes is in charge.

So why check blood glucose levels? Blood glucose monitoring provides a "snapshot" glimpse of what is happening in our bodies at one particular moment in time. Knowing what one's blood glucose level is before a meal helps with decisions about medications (particularly insulin) and provides a starting point for comparing before and after meal blood glucose levels. Knowing our blood glucose level after a meal helps us determine how particular foods and amounts of foods – and medications – affect the blood glucose. This information can help us make decisions about types and amounts of foods at future meals, as well as medication adjustment.

Blood glucose monitoring provides other important benefits. For example, checking blood glucose levels helps people with diabetes determine what is happening in our bodies. We can get in touch with when we are experiencing low blood glucose (hypoglycemia) or high blood glucose (hyperglycemia). The symptoms of low and high blood glucose can actually be very similar. Some people who have had diabetes for a while feel they know their bodies well enough to know when they are low or high. Unfortunately, symptoms of lows and highs often change over time and people who have had diabetes for many years are often less able to detect these situations. This can lead to erratic blood glucose levels because of treating a "low" that did not need treatment, or not treating a "high" that did. In other words, we're all better off knowing for sure what our blood glucose is doing by checking it regularly. Chapter 8 provides a more detailed discussion of hypoglycemia (low blood glucose).

> **Tasty Morsel (of information):** It is very common for people whose blood glucose has been running high for a while to feel low when they are not. This may happen when someone is newly diagnosed with diabetes, and their blood glucose has been extremely high for several weeks, months or even years, or someone who has been running high for a while for other reasons (illness, infection, not paying attention). In these situations, the person feels low when their blood glucose is not below 70 mg/dL, but the symptoms are real even if they occur in the 100s. As the person's average blood glucose comes down, low blood glucose symptoms will occur at lower numbers.

On more than one occasion I have thought I was low or high when I wasn't. Luckily, before treating or taking insulin, I have checked my blood glucose, discovered it was fine, and avoided unnecessary danger.

How often do we check?

For many years the recommendation that was most often heard for people with type 1 diabetes was to check at least four times a day.

Now we know that it makes sense to check more frequently than that. People with type 2 diabetes, however, tend to get mixed messages. At the very least, I recommend that people with newly diagnosed type 2 diabetes check their blood glucose levels twice a day for the first few weeks. I typically suggest a schedule for checking before and after varying meals: Monday and Thursday check before and after breakfast; Tuesday and Friday check before and after lunch; Wednesday and Saturday check before and after supper; and on Sunday choose two times to check. A before-meal check is right before you sit down to eat and an after-meal check is one-and-a-half to two hours after you start eating. The point of this schedule is to gather information for making decisions. If checking before and after lunch on work days is not realistic, it is ok to change up the schedule. You can certainly make your "lunch days" on your days off from work. It's also a good idea to check in the middle of the night occasionally. If you get up to use the bathroom, check your blood glucose. You do not need to set an alarm every night; sleep is more important than checking nightly!

The important thing is to *not* check at the same time every day. In the past, many people with type 2 diabetes were told to check fasting blood glucose levels, and the fasting blood glucose check became a way of life for many, many people. A fasting blood glucose is typically taken first thing in the morning, at least eight hours since you last ate. If you work the nightshift and your "morning" is actually in the afternoon or evening, your fasting blood glucose will be when you wake up, or after the longest period of not eating.

There has been an ongoing debate about blood glucose monitoring in type 2 diabetes. Type 2 diabetes is managed in different ways, from "diet and exercise" to pills to insulin (or other injectable medications). My suggestion is that for those who are not taking insulin or another medication that can cause low blood glucose (see Chapter 7), blood glucose monitoring can be used as a tool to "check in." After the initial few weeks of more intensive monitoring, you might cut back to once a day or a few times a week. It's a good idea to wait to cut back until your numbers are consistently in a safe and healthy (target) range.

When someone with type 2 diabetes has been checking blood glucose levels, taking medications and making consistent lifestyle behavior changes, they will eventually see their blood glucose levels stabilize. Once this happens they might choose to back off on the frequency of blood glucose monitoring, understanding two important things: 1) they will still benefit from checking blood glucose levels at least periodically, in order to detect changes that might indicate a problem or disease progression and 2) they still need to vary the timing of blood glucose checks. In other words, checking every morning when they wake up for the rest of their lives lets them know what their blood glucose level is first thing in the morning, but what about the rest of the day? In this case, I recommend checking before and after meals – and recording results accordingly – even if it's only a few times each week or month. Some people with type 2 diabetes check intensively (for example, 6 times per day) for a week and then don't check for three weeks, while others prefer to continue monitoring their blood glucose several times a day. Any of these options can work. The more we check the more we know and the better off our numbers (and health) will be overall.

People with type 1 diabetes are usually encouraged to check blood glucose levels before meals and at bedtime. The reason for this is that checking before meals helps people determine how much insulin to take for that meal. This is certainly important, and it's an excellent habit to achieve and maintain. But it's also important to know what is going on after meals, in order to make sure that the mealtime dose was effective. People who take insulin benefit from checking before *and* after meals periodically throughout the year, during pregnancy, illness, and the first couple weeks after changing insulin type or delivery method. For instance if someone switches from one type of insulin to another, or from injections to an insulin pump, checking blood glucose levels before *and* after meals helps with making necessary dose adjustments. If you are eating something new or a new combination of foods, checking your blood glucose after the meal can help you determine the most effective insulin dose for that food. If you are experiencing unexplained blood glucose levels – whether lower or higher than usual – at your usual checking times, adding a few after-meal blood glucose checks can help you solve the mystery. It is also a good idea to check before, during and after exercise, before driving a car, and when feeling signs/symptoms of high or low blood glucose.

My goal is to help people with diabetes become comfortable enough with managing their disease that they can make adjustments to their insulin doses and food choices in a confident and timely manner. With guidance and education from health care professionals and information from blood glucose monitoring, people can feel comfortable and confident making these adjustments on a day-to-day basis. Doses of medications other than insulin are not adjusted on a daily basis. Talk to your health care provider if your blood glucose levels are showing a pattern that suggests your medication dose needs to be changed.

To check or not to check

People constantly question whether or not blood glucose monitoring helps improve diabetes management. There are also ongoing discussions about whether it is more important to check blood glucose levels before or after meals. If it is not already abundantly clear that blood glucose monitoring is important, here is a recap: blood glucose monitoring provides the information necessary to determine how things are working in our daily diabetes management. Without this information we are in the dark and uninformed. Without this information we are making decisions in a random fashion. Without this information the results of our daily management are often not what we would hope for. Even people who manage their diabetes with "diet and exercise," take no medications and are relatively stable, benefit from blood glucose monitoring because they can watch for changes or disease progression. There are other ways to do this (and they will come up later), but monitoring at home, on a regular basis, puts the person with diabetes in charge. This also gives the person with diabetes the ability to detect changes earlier, which allows them to get help sooner and avoid poor health outcomes down the road.

> **Tasty Morsel (of information):** Blood glucose monitoring is expensive. For those without health insurance coverage, it may be more difficult to check blood glucose levels as frequently as is recommended. Talk to your health care professional about how to handle blood glucose monitoring if you cannot afford the strips (meters are usually free or inexpensive - it's the strips that cause the most stress on the wallet).

A little exercise…

You get to choose whether or not and how often to check your blood glucose. Use this space to jot down goals for blood glucose monitoring. Will you try something new? Will you set up a schedule?

I will start

_____

(what you're going to do)

by

_____

(put in a deadline date)

so that

_____

(what will be the outcome of your making this change?)

Fasting Blood Glucose

As mentioned earlier, the first-thing-in-the-morning reading, before you have eaten anything, is called the "fasting blood glucose." For people with type 2 diabetes, this is often the highest reading of the day, which can be extremely frustrating. I often have patients come to me and say, "My morning blood glucose is high and then it goes down all day long." People with type 2 diabetes tend to have elevated fasting blood glucose because their bodies are not working efficiently to move glucose out of the blood and into the cells. This is called insulin resistance. The cells don't recognize the insulin that their bodies make in response to glucose in the blood. As a result, the glucose cannot enter the cells. When this happens, the pancreas works even harder to make more insulin and the liver thinks it's helping out by providing glucose. The liver detects that the glucose isn't getting into the cells (but seems to miss the fact that there is plenty of glucose available), and generously (but mistakenly) starts making glucose and sending it out into the bloodstream. All this does is raise the blood glucose level higher and higher. When you haven't eaten for a long period of time, your liver thinks you are "starving" and sends glucose out. As a result the fasting blood glucose is often elevated in type 2 diabetes. Some people find that eating a healthy snack containing some carb and some protein or (healthy) fat in the evening, can help with this morning glucose. Other people take a medication to address this problem. Regular exercise is another effective approach to managing fasting blood glucose.

Another situation that has an effect on the fasting blood glucose is called the "dawn phenomenon." This is characterized by elevated fasting blood glucose that results from the body's natural surge of hormones in the "wee" hours of the morning. Hormones including cortisol, growth hormone and catecholamines (for example, adrenaline or epinephrine) work against insulin, and cause elevated fasting blood glucose levels. People who take insulin can address this problem by taking more evening insulin or by adjusting insulin pump basal doses during the challenging time period(s). This process can be very tricky; however, with practice it is possible to figure it out. Eating breakfast helps because it "turns off" these hormones and lets insulin kick in (if you still have insulin working). Even if you take insulin, eating breakfast is a good idea because once you take your insulin dose, things settle down. If you find that your blood glucose is still elevated after breakfast, you may need a higher dose of breakfast insulin. Talk to your health care provider to determine what will work best for your body.

Tasty Morsel (of information): If you are a morning exerciser and you experience the dawn phenomenon, you might consider doing what I do: I always eat breakfast before I exercise. I wake up, check my blood glucose, take insulin to correct (bring down an elevated blood glucose level), if necessary, and insulin to cover my breakfast. If it's a cardio exercise day, I take slightly less insulin than I would take on an anaerobic exercise day. Next I eat breakfast and then I exercise. This way, the insulin is working, so the dawn phenomenon stops, and there is food working, so I don't go low. By experimenting with your own food, exercise, blood glucose and medications (if you take them), you can figure out what works best for you. Be sure to work with your health care provider on this!

Another morning situation is called the "Somogyi Effect." This happens when someone sleeps through a low blood glucose event during the night and then wakes up with high blood glucose. Once again, the liver is guilty (but it's a good organ, and it's trying to help). When the liver detects that someone does not have enough glucose available (for whatever reason) it will generally kick in glucose at some point. The liver can turn glycogen (the stored form of glucose) into glucose. For those with longstanding type 1 diabetes and "hypoglycemia unawareness," this doesn't necessarily happen in time to avoid a severe low blood glucose situation (see Chapter 8). The Somogyi Effect is also called a "rebound" because a low blood glucose level rebounds and goes high. If you find that you are waking up with elevated blood glucose levels, try checking your blood glucose between 2:00 and 4:00 a.m. If you are consistently low overnight, you will need to adjust your overnight insulin dose(s) or other medication.

> **Tasty Morsel (of information)**: While checking middle of the night blood glucose levels can be extremely helpful for finding patterns and figuring out medication doses, it is important not to make this a habit. Sleep is crucial for all people, let alone those with diabetes. An occasional overnight check (or block of overnight checks) is fine, but avoid consistently sacrificing sleep for checking blood glucose levels overnight. If you really want to know what your (or your child's) blood glucose is doing overnight, consider getting a continuous

glucose monitoring system. It will alarm if you are going low, and otherwise you can look at your overnight trends in the morning.

So far, all of the crazy blood glucose situations I have mentioned are somewhat explainable. I once heard someone say that one out of every four blood glucose readings is unexplainable. And those are the extremely frustrating ones! I find myself wracking my brain to figure out why a blood glucose reading is higher than I expected. I go back and count carbs and compare that number to the insulin dose I took, I think about my activity and stress levels, and I account for the fact that some insulin gets lost in absorption. I also make sure that the insulin I'm using is good (not expired or clumping in the bottle), and those who wear an insulin pump would also check that the infusion set and pump site are good (look for crimped tubing, leaking insulin, or redness at the site). But sometimes there is just no good reason for the number on the meter, so I just accept it and move on. Take a deep, cleansing breath, distract yourself with other thoughts or tasks, but definitely move on.

Checking before vs. after meals

I hope it's pretty clear that I believe in checking blood glucose levels before *and* after meals. I have mentioned that varying the meals, themselves, is important as well. Many people who check blood glucose levels before meals only, find that they run close to or in the target range all the time. When they get their three-month average blood glucose (hemoglobin A1C) result, and it is higher than they expected, these people are often frustrated and confused. After-meal checking can reveal very different blood glucose levels than what someone is seeing fasting and before meals. This can be an indication that the body is not processing the food from the meal efficiently. The good news is that there are ways to address this problem. These solutions can include adjustments to food intake, medications and exercise. After-meal glucose checks help us determine whether or not what we are doing is working (in other words, how the food we eat affects our blood glucose), and whether or not we need to make changes. To put it another way, before-meal checks are a sort of maintenance check, and after-meal checks are a way of fine-tuning. Both are very important to managing diabetes and maintaining good health.

Blood Glucose Targets

A while back the American Diabetes Association set target blood glucose levels at 90-130 mg/dL before meals and less than 180 mg/dL after meals. More recently they have stated that diabetes management goals need to be individualized. Although I agree wholeheartedly that diabetes management goals are very personal and individual, it sometimes helps to have some idea of a healthy target for blood glucose levels. As a reminder, a before-meal blood glucose is right before a meal. I try to keep it within 30 minutes of a meal, which is a good idea if you take insulin (so you're basing your dose on a current reading). An after-meal blood glucose is approximately two hours after you start eating. The blood glucose level of someone who doesn't have diabetes may go up to 140 after a meal, but then their blood glucose level comes right back down to normal. With this in mind, a target of less than 180 is pretty liberal. I usually suggest that people use the less than 180 target when they are new to diabetes. With experience, it makes sense to bring that target down to less than 160. If you don't take insulin or a medication that causes low blood glucose, the ideal is to aim for an after-meal blood glucose of less than 140 (just like someone without diabetes).

Tasty Morsel (of information): Someone who doesn't have diabetes runs between 70 and 110 all the time. After a big meal their blood glucose might go up to 140, but it comes right back down to "normal" by the next meal. So why are the targets for someone with diabetes not the same as "normal"? I think of it as a "buffer" because we are trying to do something that our bodies would do on their own if they could. In other words, we don't yet have the ability to mimic a normally functioning body, even with all the tools we have today (but stay tuned, because scientists are working hard on finding a way to do it). Aiming for 90-130 before meals and less than 180 (160) after meals is what we have found to be a safe and healthy target, if we hit it most of the time.

Continuous Glucose Monitoring

Continuous glucose monitoring is a wonderful tool for seeing glucose trends. The continuous glucose monitoring systems available measure glucose in the interstitial fluid (the fluid that surrounds the cells in our body). These devices help people with diabetes by alerting them when glucose is trending high or low. They also display graphs of 3 to 24 hours worth of glucose levels, so you can see what happened over a period of time and make appropriate adjustments to insulin doses. Some continuous glucose monitoring systems are stand-alone devices that can be worn alongside a pump or used with injections. Other continuous glucose monitoring systems are part of an insulin pump. The trend graphs show up on the pump itself, although the pump wearer still has to be the "brains" and tell the pump how much insulin to give.

Continuous glucose monitoring (CGM) systems are helpful for gathering information on what is happening overnight, without anyone having to wake up and check a blood glucose. The machine will alarm if the glucose level is approaching a low (or high) level, and the graphs display data that can help make adjustments to insulin dosing. More and more clinics are purchasing continuous glucose monitoring systems that can be worn for three days at a time as a data collection tool. If owning your own CGM is not an option, it may be possible for you to at least wear one through your health care provider's office. CGM is constantly being improved. Stay tuned for the next generation, which will be even better than the last. Currently it is still necessary to poke fingers and check "calibration" blood glucose levels in order to keep the CGM as accurate as possible. In addition, people using CGM need to confirm a high or low reading with a fingerstick blood glucose check (before treating or taking insulin). Someday we will have a "closed loop" system – combination insulin pump and CGM - which will measure glucose levels and deliver insulin accordingly.

Ketones

When someone does not have enough insulin working, the body can't make energy from glucose. Because we must have energy to survive, the body starts breaking down fats and then proteins to produce energy. The breakdown of fats and proteins leads to a by-product called "ketones." The body works hard to excrete ketones through the urine, which can lead to dehydration. People who have ketones can get very sick, so this is a situation to take seriously. Urine or blood ketone monitoring is recommended when the blood glucose level is elevated. Please discuss guidelines with your health care provider. People with type 1 diabetes are at risk for ketones if their insulin level is not adequate for whatever reason (illness, infection, lack of insulin, extreme overeating). People with type 2 diabetes who manage their condition with insulin, and pregnant women who have gestational diabetes, may be at risk for ketones. Please ask your health care provider if you need to be concerned about this.

Ketone strips can be purchased over the counter at your local pharmacy (if they are not readily available, ask your pharmacist to order some). If you are at risk for ketones, it is a good idea to keep a bottle of ketone strips in your bathroom. These strips do expire, so make sure they are "fresh." Instructions for ketone monitoring are printed on the strip bottle. Again, it is a good idea to talk to your health care provider and make a plan for when you would need to check ketones and what to do if you have them.

Hemoglobin A1C

Hemoglobin A1C is a blood test that measures your average blood glucose over the last three months (14). That is a very simplified way of explaining it, but it's how most people understand it. I have found that blood glucose levels during the time closer to when you have the A1C drawn have more of an effect on the result. In other words, if you were on vacation for the two weeks leading up to your A1C (which invariably happens with me), it will be slightly higher than if you had been at home doing your usual thing. For the most part, however, the A1C is a wonderful tool that helps us see how we are doing with diabetes management over time. Whereas the fingerstick blood glucose gives us a peek at what's happening in one moment, a snapshot so to speak, the A1C looks at the big picture. When you get your A1C drawn, they may take the blood from your arm or from your finger. People without diabetes run between 4% and 6%, and research has shown that the closer we stay to the normal range, the less chance we have of developing diabetes-related complications (15).

The group of endocrinologists called the American Association of Clinical Endocrinologists (AACE) set the target A1C at <6.5%, while another group of diabetes professionals states it this way: keep your A1C as close to normal as possible with safety (16). In other words, if your A1C is 5.2%, but you're having frequent low blood glucose events, this is not safe. You might be better off with an A1C of 6.5 and less hypoglycemia. If your A1C is above 7% it's time to take a look at things and consider doing something different – more medication, a new medication, more exercise, smaller food portions, etc.

It is possible to have a healthy A1C, let's say 6.4%, by keeping blood glucose levels in a healthy range most of the time, or by being high some of the time and low some of the time. We also know that having blood glucose levels bounce between extremes is not healthy in the long run. Having an A1C in the 5s or even 4s, may indicate that someone is experiencing frequent lows, which is dangerous. Keeping blood glucose levels in a healthy range (see targets above) the majority of the time, leads to healthier outcomes.

> **Tasty Morsel (of information):** Research shows that if your A1C is 8% or higher, your fasting blood glucose is having the largest effect on your overall glucose management. As people tighten up their numbers and A1C comes down, this changes. For A1C levels below 8%, the after-meal glucose levels have the greatest impact on overall glucose management (17). Considering these findings, you can use your A1C level to help you make appropriate adjustments in your diabetes management.

What do we do with the numbers?

Is it starting to make sense why diabetes is "the thinking person's disease," as quoted at the beginning of the chapter? There is no reason to bother checking blood glucose levels if we are not going to use the results, and using the results requires thinking. Luckily there are tools to help us organize the results so it's a little easier to do the thinking. Blood glucose meters are sophisticated enough these days that results can be uploaded onto a computer. Numbers can be printed out in the form of a log or in fancy graphs and charts. This can be done at the health care provider's office or at home. For those who don't want to deal with technology, there are still good, old-fashioned "logbooks" where you can record your blood glucose readings. The purpose of having these numbers in writing somewhere is so you can look for patterns. A quick glance at a week's worth of blood glucose readings will tell you if you have a tendency to run high or low at particular times of the day. This practice also reminds us of the importance of gathering information (numbers) at a variety of times and not just the same time every day.

> **Tasty Morsel (of information):** Most (if not all) modern blood glucose meters have a memory, where a certain number of readings, or all readings for a certain time period, are stored. While it is certainly possible to scroll back through the memory to find past readings, they often appear in reverse chronological order (from the most recent one back), and it's very hard, if not impossible, to look for patterns this way. This is why it's so helpful to either print out or write out blood glucose records in a logbook format.

If you see a pattern and know how to fix it, go ahead and make the adjustment. That may involve changing your exercise time or amount, changing your eating habits, or adjusting your medication. ****Only adjust your medication if you take insulin and you routinely make independent adjustments to your doses. If you are new at it, if you haven't been taught how to adjust insulin doses, or if you are not** *comfortable doing so, please contact your health care provider. For all other types of medication, please contact your health care provider regarding dose adjustments.* Bring your meter, print-out, or logbook with you to every appointment. Have your health care provider take a look and make suggestions for adjustments to your diabetes management routine (if necessary). If you have made adjustments on your own, be sure to let your health care provider know.

If your daily blood glucose readings do not "match up" with your quarterly A1C level, you might have a faulty meter or strips. Check all your equipment and make sure it is working properly. More often it may be that you are checking at the same times every day, while your blood glucose is doing something different at other times. For instance, let's say that someone always checks a fasting blood glucose (first thing in the morning before eating), but never again during the day. Their fasting blood glucose readings are consistently between 110 and 135. The A1C comes back at 8%, which corresponds to a blood glucose of approximately 180 mg/dL. By checking blood glucose levels at other times of the day, specifically after meals, that person might find out that they are running in the 200s, for example, after breakfast and lunch every day. This would account for the higher A1C. Knowing what time of day we run higher (or lower), allows us to make adjustments (or get help making adjustments), so that our overall management (A1C) stays in a healthy range.

One thing we don't do with the numbers is to base our self-worth on them! If I haven't emphasized this enough, they are just numbers. Use them to make decisions, but don't stress, worry or lay blame. By checking your blood glucose you have done yourself a favor: you have become more informed. If you consistently see numbers you don't like, meet with your health care provider to figure out what you can do to change that. Stay positive, focused and motivated. *How we respond to a number is more important than the number itself.*

> **Tasty Morsel (of information):** And one more practical thing: how to get rid of used "sharps." The lancets that you use to poke your finger (and your insulin syringes and pump-related needles, if you use them) are considered "sharps," because they are sharp. The rules about disposing of sharps at home may be slightly different from state to state, so please look up your state's rules and follow them. The important thing is that you never throw used sharps directly into a trash can, sink or toilet. You can search online for "home sharps disposal in (fill in the name of your state)" and the information should come up. If not, check with your nearest board of health or public health department.

Pity Party Paragraphs

It dawned on me that readers could get this far into the book and feel like I haven't acknowledged the challenges of living with diabetes. I wholeheartedly believe that diabetes is manageable, it's not an excuse for anything, and can at times be no big deal. BUT I also acknowledge that it stinks. It's a ton of work. We didn't ask for it. It doesn't always go the way we want it to go. Despite using the smallest, finest needles on earth, injections sometimes really hurt. It doesn't go away – there's no vacation from diabetes. I have often referred to it as my "third child," because I pack for it, think about it, and take care of it. Most people without diabetes have no idea what it's like. It can be very lonely. It can affect moods and emotions. It is sometimes one huge hassle.

A little exercise:

Use this space to add any other issues you want to pity yourself about: Write them down and then crumple up the paper and throw it away (unless you think it will help you in some way).

_____

_____

_____

_____

_____

And now for a little mantra: "We acknowledge that life with diabetes has its challenges. We are not going to dwell on the challenges, but rather focus on what we can do to manage them and live healthy, abundant lives!" (Or you can make up your own mantra.)

I often hear people say, "At least you don't have ___." While that's a nice attempt to instill some perspective in a person, many (if not most) people with diabetes feel very frustrated and even angry when they hear those words. Hearing something like that can make people feel like they are not justified in their grief or anger toward having diabetes. That can even inflict guilt, which I'll get to later. On the other hand, sometimes perspective is very helpful in jumpstarting our motivation and energy to manage diabetes and take care of ourselves. Listening to a presentation or reading a book about someone else's experience (with diabetes or something else completely) can sometimes provide that perspective or even inspiration. If it would help you to read a book about someone else's struggles and how they overcame adversity, I recommend *The Gift of Fire* by Dan Caro and *Raising Lazarus* by Robert Pensack and Dwight Williams.

And that is the end of the pity party paragraphs. Let's move on.

Chapter 7
Food, Diabetes and Drugs – Oh My!

She takes her medication and eats whatever she wants.
Frequently heard from family and friends of women (and men)
with diabetes

I have type 1 diabetes, so I started taking insulin when I was first diagnosed at age seven. It's probably safe to say that most people with diabetes will take a medication at some point. Some people with type 2 diabetes manage with "diet and exercise" for a few months to several years. Some can even delay the need for medications by losing weight, staying active and making healthy food choices. Genes also play a role in all of this. Others do all the "right" things and still need several medications to keep their blood glucose in a healthy range. But most people are somewhere in the middle. They are able to make some changes in their eating and exercise habits, but still need some medication, though probably less of it than they would without the changes. Most diabetes medications have a relationship to food – either directly or indirectly. If you take diabetes medications and you are not sure which ones, please meet with your health care provider to find out exactly which medications you take, how they work, and what the possible side effects are.

Tasty Morsel (of information): The normally functioning pancreas produces and secretes insulin constantly throughout the day and night, and then whenever there is food on board. There are triggers in the body that tell the pancreas when insulin is needed. In someone with diabetes this system does not work properly. The purpose of managing diabetes is to achieve blood glucose levels as close to normal as possible, as much of the time as possible, in a safe way. Most of the time this requires medication.

Understanding your diabetes medications can make it easier and more likely that you will take them. One study showed that one in three people with diabetes does not take their insulin as prescribed (18). It would not be surprising if this is true for other diabetes medications as well. People miss taking their medications for many reasons. Some people forget to take medications; others are not convinced they need the medication or have preconceived notions about taking medications. Some people cannot afford their medications and some people fear side effects from diabetes medication or addiction to them. Some people feel as if medications are running their lives, or they have a lack of support. Again, having a thorough knowledge of which medications you take, why they have been prescribed for you, and how they work can alleviate many of those concerns.

There are many myths related to taking insulin. Some people believe that taking insulin means they have "worse diabetes." Sometimes people think that if they go on insulin, they will be on it for life. Although people with type 1 diabetes need insulin for life, many people with type 2 diabetes take insulin during hospitalizations and/or for short periods of time. Insulin may be necessary during illness, surgery, or infection, and not during other times. In some instances, people with type 2 diabetes may lose a substantial amount of weight and find they no longer need to take insulin.

There are several reasons why people don't want to start taking insulin. William Polonsky and Richard Jackson (19) discussed six factors that play into people's reluctance to take insulin: 1) perceived loss of control over one's life, 2) lack of confidence in handling the demands of insulin, 3) personal failure, 4) perception that one's diabetes is getting worse, 5) fear of injections/needles, and 6) perceived lack of benefits from taking insulin.

It is important to know that managing diabetes with insulin is doable and, if necessary to achieve and maintain a healthy life, you can do it too! With the help of health care providers and a support system, anyone can gain the confidence to handle insulin. If your health care provider looks you in the eye one day and tells you that your body needs insulin, please remember that it is not because you are a failure. It's because your current medications or management approach have failed *you*, and it's time to try something else. Type 2 diabetes is a progressive disease, and over time many people need to start insulin - not because it's "worse," but because it has changed. A lot of people fear needles/injections. Luckily, insulin syringes and insulin pens have very short and thin needles. Ask your health care provider to show you how small they are. People often think that once they start insulin bad things will happen. It is actually the opposite - not taking insulin when it is needed can lead to poor health outcomes. Even though you may not take insulin right now, the information on the following pages could be helpful if you ever do need it, or if you know someone who takes insulin.

Insulin

Insulin is a vital hormone that is made by the beta cells of the pancreas. Insulin's job is to take glucose out of the blood and into the cells. When someone with a normally functioning pancreas eats food, it gets broken down into glucose. The pancreas makes insulin in response to the rise in glucose in the bloodstream. Insulin hooks up with "receptors" on the walls of liver, muscle and fat cells throughout the body. Once the insulin is hooked up, channels open and allow glucose to get inside the cells. Glucose is then used by the cells to make energy. We need this energy to perform every imaginable function – from breathing and thinking to walking, working and even sleeping!

Type 1 diabetes is an autoimmune disorder, where antibodies kill off the beta cells of the pancreas, because they see them as "foreign." This means that people with type 1 diabetes cannot make insulin and therefore have to take it from an outside source in order to survive. Meanwhile for people with type 2 or gestational diabetes either insulin isn't used effectively, or their bodies don't make enough insulin. Very often, people with type 2 diabetes start with "insulin resistance," which means the cells don't recognize the insulin they make. Because the insulin can't hook up on the receptors, the channels do not open and the glucose can't get into the cells. The pancreas responds to this situation by working overtime to make more insulin, trying to get enough out there to make things work. People can get by for months or even years, but during this time the pancreas is actually burning itself out. This is one of the reasons why it is so important to diagnose type 2 diabetes as early as possible. As a result of all this hard work, the pancreas eventually may not be able to keep up and many people with type 2 diabetes end up needing to take insulin from the outside at some point. I tell every patient with newly diagnosed type 2 (or gestational) diabetes that if, one day, their health care provider looks them in the eye and says, "you need insulin," take it! Insulin is good. I would not be alive if it weren't for insulin.

The key is to take the right amount of the right type(s) of insulin, at the right times. Insulin has a terrible reputation for making people gain weight; however, it is possible to take insulin and not gain weight. It's excess food that makes people gain weight, not insulin. The trick is to eat the right amount of food for your body – and exercise! If you eat more calories than your body needs – or than you burn off – and take insulin to cover it, you will gain weight, just like someone without diabetes. Insulin is a "storage hormone": it helps your body to store unused glucose as fat, which is why taking more insulin than you need (also known as eating more food than you need) equals weight gain. Work with your health care provider to come up with an insulin plan that fits your eating and exercise plan.

When it comes to insulin, we have truly come a long way. Michael Bliss wrote a book called *The Discovery of Insulin*, which details what was happening for people with diabetes before, during and after insulin was first isolated, extracted and then injected into humans. Since the first insulin became commercially available in 1922, we have had several different sources and types of insulin. We started out with insulin from cows and pigs (and many other creatures), and now we have synthetic insulin that is made to be exactly the same as human insulin (luckily, no humans are sacrificed in the process). We currently have insulin that works faster and insulin that lasts longer than insulins of the past. These discoveries have allowed those of us who use insulin to fine-tune our diabetes management.

The first type of insulin, called Regular insulin, was considered "short-acting." Many years after Regular was first made, scientists added protein to it and created NPH. The added protein made it work longer. Over the years scientists also added zinc to Regular insulin, which gave us the lente insulins. In the 1980s scientists figured out how to make "human" (synthetic) insulin, and after a few years, the manufacturing of animal-based insulin ended in the United States. At that time the two biggest insulin manufacturers produced Regular and NPH insulin in a "human" version. Lilly named their "human" insulin Humulin, and NovoNordisk named theirs Novolin. For instance, someone might take Humulin R (Regular) and Humulin N (NPH).

Several years later rapid-acting insulin analogs were created. Lilly named theirs Humalog® and NovoNordisk named theirs NovoLog®. These names have caused quite a bit of confusion for people. There have even been mix-ups at the pharmacy, where people have gotten the wrong type of insulin. Be sure that you know exactly what type of insulin you take, and what brand. When you pick up your prescriptions, check the labels and the vials to be sure you got what you were supposed to get. More recently another insulin manufacturer, Sanofi, brought us Apidra®, the third of the rapid-acting insulins. Currently, we also have two long-acting insulin analogs available: Lantus® and Levemir®. Long-acting insulin is taken once or twice a day and serves as a background dose that works around the clock. Rapid-acting insulin is taken before meals.

If you take insulin, it's very important to know when it starts working, when it peaks, and when it is gone. Rapid-acting insulins start working in 10 to 15 minutes, peak in 90 minutes, and are gone in approximately three to four hours. These types of insulin basically cover a meal: their action peaks while the blood glucose is highest from the food that was just eaten. Long-acting insulins work from 12 to 24 hours, although the longest of them probably only work for about 20 to 22 hours. New insulins are being developed all the time, so stay tuned! And if you take a "pre-mixed" insulin such as "70/30," 75/25," or "50/50," talk to your provider to find out when they are working and what precautions you need to take.

> **Tasty Morsel (of information):** When I was eight my parents sent me to diabetes camp to learn how to give myself insulin injections. This is no joke. Although they most likely also sent me to camp to have fun and meet friends with diabetes, this was not the priority. They sent me to learn how to take "shots." Nowadays, kids are not forced to self-inject insulin at an early age. In fact, now we encourage kids to begin giving injections only when they are ready. And they will let us know when they are ready. Diabetes camp is a place for kids with diabetes to have fun in a safe environment, where everyone is checking blood glucose levels, taking insulin and counting carbs – even the counselors. Kids play games and do crazy, fun things while learning about diabetes. The most important lesson is that diabetes doesn't stop them from doing anything in life.

Insulin is taken through the subcutaneous (fatty) tissue, and there are a few different ways to deliver it. Insulin comes in vials and pens. Syringes are used to draw insulin from a vial (bottle) and inject it into the body. In the United States, the concentration of insulin is called "U-100," which means there are 100 units in a cubic centimeter or milliliter. This is a way to measure the concentration of insulin, and the most important thing to know is that U-100 syringes go with U-100 insulin. In other countries the concentration may be different.

Insulin pens hold up to 300 units of insulin. They are a convenient way to carry insulin, because it's all in one and doesn't require a vial and syringe. You connect a needle to the end of the pen, dial up the dose and inject. Some people reuse needles at home, and it's important to know that pen needles need to be changed at least after two to three uses to avoid problems. If the pen needle is left on the pen, insulin can crystallize inside the needle. This can cause a blockage, and the next time you try to push the plunger it can break the entire mechanism, rendering the pen useless.

> **Tasty Morsel (of information):** If you inject insulin by pen or syringe, you need to know about injection sites. You can basically inject wherever you have some fatty tissue. We call this subcutaneous tissue, which is just below your skin. Common injection sites include the abdomen, backs of the arms, legs, buttocks, and hips. It is important to not only rotate among the sites, but within the sites as well, in order to preserve them over time. Injecting insulin into the same area can cause damage to the tissue, which can eventually lead to poor absorption of the insulin. You may have noticed that pen needles and syringe needles come in a variety of lengths. The distance from outside your skin to the subcutaneous layer is not far at all, and so shorter and shorter needles have become available. The best thing to do is try them out! Use a needle length that makes you feel comfortable, and pay attention to blood glucose patterns. If everything is looking the way you want it to, stick with that length. If you are running low, take less insulin (talk to your provider about how much), and if you are running consistently high, consider trying a different needle length.

Insulin Pumps

Another name for insulin pump is CSII (continuous subcutaneous insulin infusion). This is the closest we can get to mimicking a functioning pancreas at this time, although many "artificial pancreases" are being studied. An insulin pump involves an "infusion set," which has a catheter (tube) that is inserted into your fatty tissue (same places where you can give an injection). The infusion set is connected to tubing, which is connected to a syringe that holds insulin inside the pump. There are also some insulin pumps that do not have tubing, which may be a very appealing alternative.

Pumps deliver insulin in a very effective way – continuous pulsing throughout the day and night. As a result, only one type of insulin is used in the pump: rapid-acting insulin. Those who took long-acting insulin (Lantus® or Levemir®) injections would stop using that kind altogether when they go on a pump. The pump is programmed to deliver insulin 24 hours per day (basal dose) and then every time you eat or need to correct a high blood glucose you push buttons to give a bolus dose. The only drawback to having fast-acting insulin in the pump is that if the pump were to stop functioning, the insulin currently working in the body would run out very quickly.

Typically, pump wearers find they use less insulin than when they took injections. One challenge with insulin pumps, however, is that it is very easy to "dial up" for a snack. Any time you want to eat, you don't have to think about drawing up and injecting insulin, so it can lead to less healthy eating habits. It's easy enough to "cover" food with insulin, to keep blood glucose levels (and A1Cs – see Chapter 6) in a healthy range. While it is definitely important to do so, the downside is this practice can lead to weight gain and can also contribute to high cholesterol, high blood pressure and other health problems that go along with weight gain. Once again, it's a matter of making choices. If you choose to have an occasional splurge, by all means take enough insulin to cover it! Just be aware of how often this happens and if it starts becoming a habit, it's time to make a change.

> **Tasty Morsel (of information):** If you wear a pump and find you are slipping into this type of habitual eating and dosing, try taking off the pump for a while and going

back to injections. Being on injections could provide the reminder you need – to make a healthy choice – each time you feel like snacking on extra calories. It is ok to take a break from an insulin pump for other reasons as well. Work with your health care provider to determine how to dose insulin (and what types to use) if you decide to go on injections.

People often wonder if there is a certain amount of time that must go by between being diagnosed with diabetes - or between starting on insulin - and starting on a pump. The answer is a qualified "no." There is no magic number of injections someone has to give before going on an insulin pump, although it's important to know how to draw up and inject insulin in case the pump were to malfunction. It is also important to know how and be willing to monitor blood glucose levels frequently and count carbs before starting on an insulin pump. I've sometimes wondered if the day will come when people are put on pumps before they ever take injections. It could happen! But insulin pumps are not for everyone, so those who are not interested don't have to worry that they will be forced to use one.

There is no magic age for wearing an insulin pump either. I know of two-year-olds on insulin pumps, and there may be even younger kids pumping out there. This means, of course, that the parents are in charge. The parents (or some adult person) are the ones who program the pump doses, change the infusion sets, and calculate how many carbs are being eaten. We now have continuous glucose monitoring (see Chapter 6), which can be combined with some insulin pumps.

In Chapter 2 we discussed the effect of fat, especially high-fat "combo" foods, on blood glucose. Meals like pizza, many Mexican dishes and many Chinese dishes are high in both carb and fat. Pumps are ideal for handling these situations because you can actually program them to deliver some insulin right away (before or as you eat) and some over time. For instance, if your blood glucose is 180 mg/dL and you are about to have pizza, you could take half of your mealtime insulin right away and half over the next two hours (the amount of time is determined by trial and error). That way you have insulin working on both the pre-meal blood glucose and the carb (crust) in the pizza. The remaining insulin can cover the effect of the fat (cheese, oil, sausage, etc.). If, on the other hand, your blood glucose was 80 mg/dL before the meal, you might take the entire dose over time and none of it before the meal.

So far the pumps we have available are considered an "open loop" system. This means that the person wearing the pump - or their caregiver - has to be the brains. We have to check and enter blood glucose levels, calculate and enter carb servings, program doses, and generally manage the pump. The ultimate goal with insulin pumps is the "closed loop" system: one that monitors glucose levels, determines the appropriate dose, and delivers it. This type of system is currently being tested and will one day be a reality.

Without a pump, you can still tweak the timing of your mealtime insulin, somewhat. I recommend that people take their fast-acting insulin *after* a high-fat meal. Another trick is to inject the fast-acting insulin into a more slowly absorbing site. The arms and abdomen absorb insulin more quickly, while the thighs and buttocks absorb insulin more slowly.

> **Tasty Morsel (of information):** Taking rapid-acting insulin 10-20 minutes before meals helps keep after-meal blood glucose levels in a healthier range. For the average, non-high-fat meal, therefore, try to make it a habit to inject (deliver) insulin 10-20 minutes before eating. I base the amount of time on my current (pre-meal) blood glucose. If I'm low, I take the insulin and start eating immediately. If I'm in my target range, I take

it 10-15 minutes before eating, and if I'm high I take it about 20 minutes before eating. Be careful not to take your pre-meal insulin and then get distracted with a project. Another recommendation is to avoid taking insulin at home for a meal that will be eaten elsewhere; don't set yourself up for having too much time go by between rapid-acting insulin and a meal. Those who are not sure how much they will eat at a meal may need to take insulin after they start eating - or even after they are finished - in order to determine how much insulin they need.

Since we started taking insulin according to what we're about to eat – some people have gotten into the habit of "eating whatever they want." This is also true of many people who take other diabetes medications. It is important to remember that medication is just one part of the balancing act in diabetes management. Making healthy food choices and exercising (and managing stress) are equally important. Taking medication and then eating "whatever we want" can lead to out-of-target (high) blood glucose levels and weight gain, which can lead to blood vessel damage.

> **Tasty Morsel (of information):** Microvascular complications are those complications that involve very small blood vessels. This includes eye disease (the blood vessels in the back, or retina, of the eye); kidney disease; and nerve disease. Macrovascular complications involve large vessels and include heart disease and stroke. The point of managing diabetes is to avoid developing any of these complications by keeping all the blood vessels healthy.

As mentioned earlier, taking more insulin than we need, usually because we are eating more food than we need can lead to significant weight gain. If we "eat whatever we want" and take insulin to "cover" the extra food, we will gain weight. People with both type 1 and type 2 diabetes can experience weight gain. Being overweight, in turn, contributes to other health problems including high cholesterol, high blood pressure, heart disease, stroke, and cancer. It can also contribute to depression. Taking the right amount of insulin and eating the right amount of food for our bodies are, therefore, important for more reasons than just managing blood glucose.

Many people resist going on insulin for a variety of reasons. Sometimes it's the health care provider who doesn't encourage people to take insulin and other times the resistance comes from the person who needs the insulin. Some people resist insulin because of their job. For instance, people who have a commercial driver's license (CDL) know that taking insulin means jumping through several hoops to get a special consideration for their CDL. Many people with diabetes mistakenly think that insulin is the cause of problems like losing limbs and going blind. This is not true! Not taking insulin when you need it causes these devastating problems. I have had patients tell me they can't go on insulin because their spouse will be mad at them. It is very helpful to figure out what you think about insulin. Get to the bottom of it, so that you can work through it and be ok with insulin if you need it someday. It may help to talk to your loved ones and explain to them that insulin is good and necessary. Bring them to an appointment and have your health care professional explain it, if that is more effective.

Many people feel that having to take insulin means they have failed. Diabetes professionals are working hard to get rid of this misconception. To reiterate, people with type 1 diabetes need insulin from the start, because their pancreas no longer makes it. People with latent autoimmune diabetes in adults (LADA) typically start taking insulin within six years of being diagnosed. Type 2 diabetes, on the other hand, is a progressive disorder. Some people start out managing type 2 diabetes with "diet and exercise." Most people with type 2 take metformin (more on this momentarily). There are several oral medications for type 2 diabetes and most people progress to needing some combination of them. Many people with type 2 diabetes, despite checking blood glucose levels, taking their pills and even exercising, progress to needing insulin at some point. Again, this is not failure, this is normal disease progression. Some people are diagnosed with type 2 diabetes and then discover they need insulin very early on. As mentioned in Chapter 1, this is sometimes called LADA (latent autoimmune diabetes in adults, which some providers call "type 1.5" diabetes). The only way someone would go from type 2 to type 1 diabetes is if they were given the wrong diagnosis at the outset. Type 2 diabetes does not progress to type 1 diabetes (remember, type 1 diabetes is an autoimmune disorder and type 2 is not). Those with type 2 diabetes who take insulin still have type 2 diabetes.

Some people insist that they cannot or will not take insulin. This may be related to a fear of needles or something else completely. You may want to do some soul searching and figure out how you feel about your health, your future, and insulin. If insulin becomes something you need, I promise that you *can* take it (the needles are tiny, the technique is easy, and with time you can get used to it). Without insulin (if you need it), you run the risk of devastating complications from high blood glucose levels. Sometimes we have certain ideas or thoughts about health-related topics. These are called health beliefs, and we may not even be aware of them. They might have originated with earlier experiences or beliefs that were passed down through generations, or maybe even societal beliefs. When I was pregnant, I knew I would need to double, if not triple the amount of insulin I took before becoming pregnant. However, when it came time to take that much insulin, I was filled with thoughts of "this can't be good for me." I honestly don't know where those thoughts came from. I have never had a negative opinion of or experience with insulin. Luckily, I pushed past those feelings, took the insulin I (and my babies) needed and had healthy outcomes.

> **Tasty Morsel (of information):** If you struggle with the thought of taking one more medication, try this: Don't think of insulin as a medication/drug. Think of it as a life-sustaining liquid that your body needs to do its best work. You could even call it the "internal secretion" as they did before insulin was named in 1921!

A little exercise:

Write down what insulin means to you (include any insulin-related concerns for your spouse or family members that would/do affect you if you took/take insulin):

_____

_____

_____

_____

_____

Write down ways you can work through any negative feelings or concerns you may have about insulin:

_____

_____

_____

_____

_____

Biguanides

Metformin (Glucophage) is a medication that most people with type 2 diabetes take. Metformin tells the liver not to send extra glucose into the bloodstream. This is an important job because the majority of people with type 2 diabetes have "insulin resistance." This is a situation where the insulin that the person's body makes is not used properly so the glucose can't get out of the blood and into the cells. As a result, the liver tries to help out by sending in more glucose. All this does is raise the blood glucose level even higher. This problem tends to occur overnight, so people with type 2 diabetes sometimes find that their fasting (first thing in the morning) blood glucose is the highest of the day. Metformin helps to lower the fasting blood glucose.

Some of the common side effects of metformin include gas, cramping, bloating, nausea and diarrhea. The good news, however, is that these side effects usually subside within a week or two. If you take metformin with food and take it every day as directed, you are much less likely to experience these side effects. Metformin is started at a lower dose and increased as needed over time. With the exception of a handful of people who just cannot tolerate metformin, those patients who complain of ongoing side effects are usually taking it without food, inconsistently, or their dose was not increased slowly. There are also combination drugs that contain both metformin and another diabetes medication. Check with your health care provider to see if you take metformin or a metformin combination drug.

> **Tasty Morsel (of information):** If you are sick or are scheduled for a medical or surgical procedure, you may need to stop taking your metformin (or metformin

combination drug). Metformin is cleared from your body through your kidneys, so if there is any chance you could become dehydrated, you don't want metformin to back up in your system. Be sure to follow whatever instructions you are given by your health care professional.

Sulfonylureas and Meglitinides

Sulfonylureas and meglitinides are also medications used to treat type 2 diabetes. In fact, sulfonylureas are the oldest class of type 2 medications and meglitinides are a newer version of medications that work similarly to sulfonylureas. Sulfonylureas work by telling the pancreas to secrete more insulin. There are several different names of pills that fall into these categories, so be sure to check with your health care provider to see if you are taking one. It is very important to eat at regular times when taking sulfonylureas. When the insulin kicks in, it needs some food to work on. If there is no or not enough food available, hypoglycemia (low blood glucose, which is discussed in the next chapter) will occur. Meglitinides also tell the pancreas to secrete insulin, but they do it in a more controlled fashion. Meglitinides are taken right before meals and they work over a shorter time (usually the course of the meal), while the food is working. For this reason, there is less risk of hypoglycemia with meglitinides, although it can still happen.

Alpha-Glucosidase Inhibitors

Alpha-glucosidase inhibitors are type 2 diabetes pills that stop the body from breaking down carbohydrates, and this helps to lower the blood glucose level. These medications can cause pretty severe gas and cramping. If someone taking one of these medications has a low blood glucose level, they need to treat it with pure glucose in the form of glucose tablets or gel, because the body is unable to use things like white sugar or orange juice. This is a very important precaution to know about if you take an alpha-glucosidase inhibitor. Check with your health care provider to see if you are taking one of these drugs.

Thiazolidinediones (TZDs)

These type 2 diabetes pills address insulin resistance, but in a different way from metformin. TZDs actually go in and work directly on the cells, specifically the receptors that hook up the insulin. They help the receptors start recognizing insulin again. This "reprogramming" of the cells takes several weeks to get going, so people who take TZDs often don't see an effect for 4 to 6 weeks. TZDs don't really have a relationship with food, although they can cause edema (swelling), which can be mistaken for weight gain. It is often described as more of a redistribution of weight.

GLP-1 Mimetics

In the normally functioning body, the gut has hormones that respond to the first bite of food by telling the pancreas to make insulin. We now know that in people with type 2 diabetes, these gut hormones don't work as well as they should. Byetta, Victoza® and Bydureon are injectable type 2 diabetes medications that mimic GLP-1, which is one of these gut hormones. GLP-1 mimetics help the pancreas produce insulin, but they work only if there is glucose in the blood. This means that, on their own, these drugs do not cause hypoglycemia. Byetta can cause nausea, however, and it needs to be taken within 60 minutes of the two largest meals each day. Victoza® works like Byetta, but is taken only once a day, while Bydureon is taken only once a week. In addition to telling the pancreas to produce insulin, GLP-1 mimetics suppress glucagon, a hormone that raises blood glucose, and then go to the brain and send a message of fullness, so the person doesn't eat as much.

Finally, they slow gastric emptying, so the person feels full longer. As a result, some people lose weight when taking these medications. Pharmaceutical companies are continuously working on newer versions of these medications.

> **Tasty Morsel (of information):** Like insulin, glucagon is a hormone made by the pancreas. Where insulin lowers blood glucose, glucagon's job is to tell the liver to break down stored glucose (glycogen) and send it out into the bloodstream. Therefore, glucagon plays a role in raising the blood glucose level when it is low. With diabetes, however, glucagon does not work the way it is supposed to. It tends to go to work after meals, when there is already enough glucose circulating, and just contributes to a higher blood glucose level.

DPP-IV Inhibitors

While the gut hormones are doing their job telling the pancreas to make insulin and so on, there is an enzyme that is mobilized to inactivate those gut hormones. This creates a balance in the system so that the right amount of insulin is secreted. Unfortunately, with type 2 diabetes, that enzyme, called "dipeptidyl peptidase-IV or DPP-IV," works too fast. This is part of the reason why the gut hormones are less effective. A relatively new class of drugs, the DPP-IV inhibitors stop the enzyme from shutting down the gut hormones so fast. The DPP-IV inhibitors currently available in the United States are Januvia®, Onglyza®, and Tradjenta®.

Symlin

In someone who doesn't have diabetes, the pancreas makes insulin and amylin at the same time. Amylin is a hormone that suppresses glucagon and makes people feel full. In people with type 1 diabetes, the pancreas does not produce insulin or amylin. Symlin, a synthetic form of amylin, works by helping people feel full after they eat, and suppressing glucagon. Symlin can cause nausea, so it's helpful to start with a lower dose and work up to the highest dose needed. Insulin doses have to be adjusted because of an increased risk of hypoglycemia. Talk to your health care provider if you are interested in learning more about Symlin.

SGLT-2 Inhibitors

A new class of type 2 diabetes medications is called sodium glucose co-transporter 2 (SGLT2) inhibitors. These drugs work by increasing the excretion of glucose in the urine. Canagliflozin (Invokana) and dapagliflozin (Farxiga) are the first two drugs in this class. As with any medication, talk to your health care provider to see if this is an appropriate option for you.

Chapter 8
Hypoglycemia

Hypoglycemia, or low blood glucose, is sometimes called a "low," a "hypo," or a "reaction." Sometimes hypoglycemia has also been referred to as "insulin shock." Hypoglycemia means there is not enough glucose circulating in the bloodstream, or the blood glucose level is too "low." Hypoglycemia is defined as a blood glucose level below 70 mg/dL. People who take insulin, sulfonylureas, meglitinides (or any medication that contains a sulfonylurea or meglitinide), or Symlin are at risk for hypoglycemia. Many of the pills used to manage type 2 diabetes do not cause hypoglycemia. Check with your health care provider to see which type of medication you take and if it causes hypoglycemia.

> **Tasty morsel (of information):** In many/most cases, hypoglycemia is a predictable event. Some people fear low blood glucose to such an extent that they do not keep their blood glucose levels in a healthy range. This does not have to be the case!

A little exercise:

Get in touch with your feelings about hypoglycemia. Do you fear low blood glucose? Do you find it annoying? Write down whatever comes to mind when you think about low blood glucose:

_____

_____

_____

_____

_____

Now write down ways you can work through these feelings and not let hypoglycemia get in your way:

_____

_____

_____

_____

_____

Hypoglycemia has a variety of different signs and symptoms. If you are relatively new to diabetes, the most common symptom is shakiness. Unfortunately, signs and symptoms of hypoglycemia can change over time. Those who have had diabetes for many years may tell you that they don't get shaky anymore. Sometimes they develop completely different signs and symptoms and sometimes they experience "hypoglycemia unawareness," which means they do not feel their lows at all. Some people need to pay closer attention to subtle signs and symptoms of low blood glucose.

I am one of those people whose symptoms have changed over time. I can't tell you how many years it's been since I experienced shakiness as a low symptom. For a while I could tell I was low because the lights would shake or flash. I once had a nurse practitioner who explained that if you are set to go out and you just can't leave the house – you're wandering around in a daze or can't find your keys (on the counter) – check your blood glucose because you are probably low. Most recently, my low symptoms are subtle enough that they are hard to explain, but fortunately I still know when I'm low. Sometimes I get a headache or even feel nauseated; sometimes I'm grumpy or snap easily; sometimes, believe it or not, I *yawn* repeatedly. The most important thing

I've learned is to really pay attention to the little clues that something is not right and *check my blood glucose.*

> **Tasty Morsel of Information**: *Symptoms* are what you feel or experience and s*igns* are what someone else looks for. It's a good idea to know these and let others know. For example, I once had a camper at diabetes camp whose mother alerted me that her daughter's left eye drooped when she was low. That was helpful to know in case that camper went low during an activity. While this girl's symptoms (for example, shakiness) may have been masked by her excitement for the activity, I would be able to detect her low sooner and help her treat it.

Other symptoms include, but are certainly not limited to, headache, blurred vision, weakness, hunger, sweating, and confusion. Signs of hypoglycemia include pale skin, irritability, changes in personality (for example, a typically serious person may get silly, a typically happy person may get grumpy, or a typically talkative person may get quiet), combativeness, confusion, and unresponsiveness. If you know someone with diabetes, ask them if they are at risk for low blood glucose. If so, ask them what their signs and symptoms are, so you can be aware if they need help (or a gentle reminder to check their blood glucose and/or eat something). Occasionally people can get cranky when they are low and refuse to treat the low. If you know someone who reacts in this way, you may have to make a plan (when they are not low) about how this type of situation will be handled.

> **Tasty Morsel (of information):** Severe hypoglycemia, where the person is unresponsive, unconscious or having a seizure, is considered a medical emergency. This person is unable to take treatment by mouth and emergency personnel may need to be called. Some

people keep a Glucagon Emergency Kit handy, which can be used by someone who has been taught how. Glucagon Emergency Kits can be obtained with a prescription from your local pharmacy (they may have to order it for you). These kits have expiration dates, so they can be kept in the refrigerator until they expire, and then they need to be replaced.

Hypoglycemia is getting its own chapter because it is a big deal, relates directly to food and eating, and can cause problems for people. Hypoglycemia occurs when there is too much insulin working for what the body needs. This can occur for a variety of reasons:

- Too much insulin/medication taken
- Not enough food eaten
- Extra or unplanned exercise performed

Someone can take too much insulin by accident. A common mistake is to draw up the right dose of the wrong insulin. For example, if someone usually takes 30 units of long-acting insulin, but they mistakenly drew up 30 units of rapid-acting insulin. The long-acting insulin would have worked over the course of many hours, while the rapid-acting insulin will now kick in (with a vengeance!) in about 20 minutes and peak in 90 minutes. This is another reason why it's so important to be familiar with medication labels - know what each type of insulin is called, how it works, and what the bottle/label looks like. Some people come up with little systems for storing insulin vials so they take the right one at the right time. If this does happen to you, stay calm and act quickly to consume enough carbohydrate to compensate for the insulin. If this is not possible, or if there is any question regarding your safety, call 911 immediately.

Another set-up for hypoglycemia is taking the usual insulin/sulfonylurea dose and then not eating as much food as the dose requires. In this case the person would have all this insulin working and not enough food for it to work on. This might also happen if someone took their usual insulin dose and ate their usual meal and then decided to join a friend for a long walk on the spur of the moment. They would have the right amount of insulin for the amount of food they ate, but the extra (unplanned) activity would lower the blood glucose level.

Our brains need glucose to survive. The brain cannot get energy from any other source (whereas the rest of our body could live off of fat and protein for a while if it had to). As a result, some of the symptoms of low blood glucose are messages that come directly from the brain. The brain's way of saying, "Hey, I need some glucose, here!" may be through a headache or vision changes, or in extreme circumstances even a seizure or loss of consciousness. Since the brain is the control center for the entire body, we really don't want to mess with it. Keep your brain happy by providing enough glucose for it to do its job!

If you suspect your blood glucose is low, check first before treating so you can 1) confirm that you are low and 2) prevent the situation of eating/drinking unnecessary calories. Believe it or not, the signs and symptoms of hypoglycemia can be very similar to (and sometimes the same as) high blood glucose - fatigue, blurred vision, hunger, headache, and mood swings can be symptoms of both high and low blood glucose. If your blood glucose is actually high (when you feel low), you probably don't want to consume something sweet. On the other hand, if you are experiencing symptoms of a low blood glucose, and you don't have access to your blood glucose monitoring equipment, it's safer to just treat the low. And the best way to prevent hypoglycemia in the first place, is by routinely checking blood glucose levels (see Chapter 6).

A blood glucose below 70 mg/dL is considered low; however, some people feel low when their blood glucose is in the 80s, 90s or even 100s. This can happen especially if the person's blood glucose levels have been running high for a while and their body got used to having all that glucose around. When the blood glucose gets down to the normal range (70-110), their body panics and thinks they are out of glucose. As the average glucose level comes down, this will subside and the person will feel low when they are actually low (less than 70). I recommend eating a hard candy if you feel low but are not actually low: it won't affect your blood glucose level significantly, but it can make the low feeling go away.

If you have not yet experienced a low blood glucose

If you are brand new to diabetes (or know someone who is), you may not have experienced a "low" yet. I strongly recommend frequent blood glucose monitoring if you take a medication that may cause hypoglycemia. If you feel any of the symptoms of hypoglycemia (see earlier section), check your blood glucose right away, if possible, and confirm that you are low and then make a mental note of what you are feeling. This is also important if you live with someone who has diabetes. The first several times they complain of any of the symptoms (or you notice signs) of a low, have them check their blood glucose and then you will know what to look for in the future. I still recommend checking to confirm a low even after you feel confident you know what your signs and symptoms are. Invariably, you will find yourself in situations where you can't check first, and it will be helpful to know what a low feels like. When in doubt, or if you don't have your monitoring supplies handy, go ahead and treat it as a low. It is more dangerous to not treat a low that is really occurring than it is to over treat what you think is a low, but is actually a normal or high level.

Another time when someone could feel low and have a blood glucose reading in the normal (or even slightly high) range, is if their blood glucose level is dropping rapidly. For this reason, it's a good idea to re-check the blood glucose level in 5 to 15 minutes, especially if the symptoms do not subside This can happen during strenuous activity or because a medication has "kicked in."

One issue with hypoglycemia is that you might want to eat until the feeling goes away. For some people, hypoglycemia is one of their "triggers" for overeating. All you actually need to raise your blood glucose level is approximately 15 grams of carbohydrate. However, depending on how much insulin you have working or when your next meal will be, you might actually need more calories to "hold you over." A good rule of thumb is to treat the low immediately with a pure carbohydrate source (orange juice, glucose tablets, hard candy) and then follow that with a more substantial snack if your next meal is more than one hour away. If you are low and are just about to eat a meal, another idea is to eat a carbohydrate food first, e.g., a roll or potato or piece of fruit. On the other hand, if you are low and are in the middle of a hike, cleaning the house, or other strenuous activity, follow the "low treatment" with a snack that contains more substance. Some crackers and cheese or a piece of fruit and a handful of nuts would probably do the trick.

Tasty morsel (of information): Fifteen grams of carbohydrate raises the blood glucose approximately 50 mg/dL. Keeping this in mind, here are some examples of effective hypoglycemia treatments:

- ½ cup (4 oz.) orange juice (the 4 to 6-oz. juice boxes work great!)
- 3 or 4 glucose tablets (sold at pharmacy counters)
- ½ of a standard banana
- 1 cup (8 oz.) fat-free milk
- hard candy (check nutrition label for amount needed to equal 15 grams of carb)

Because it is tempting to *eat until the feeling goes away*, the best thing to do is get the blood glucose level up fast. Fat takes much longer to break down in the body than carbohydrate. In addition, not much of the fat turns into glucose in the bloodstream. Therefore, it's helpful to avoid treating hypoglycemia with high-fat food items. Although it's tempting, when you're feeling this way, avoid eating chocolate bars, ice cream, fudge, etc. They will take longer to "kick in," which makes you more likely to overeat, and they will shoot the blood glucose level way up and keep it up for several hours later. In combination foods that contain both carbohydrate and fat, the fat can slow down the glucose-raising effect of the carbohydrate.

Some additional ideas for fast hypoglycemia treatment include jelly beans, Skittles®, cake frosting, maple syrup, honey, and regular soda. I try to stick to items that I will not want to snack on otherwise. Jelly beans work for me: I have found that one regular jelly bean raises my blood glucose approximately 10 mg/dL, so I can take as many as I need to get back up to my target, which is 100 mg/dL. For example, if my blood glucose is 60 mg/dL, I will eat four jelly beans. If I am in the middle of something more strenuous, like a walk, I will eat more. I, for one, am not likely to overeat jelly beans, but if jelly beans are a personal weakness, choose something else! And remember that all jelly beans are not equal, so do some experimenting.

Tasty Morsel (of information): If you live with or are frequently around children who like sweet treats, be sure to explain that your "low treatment" (whatever that is) is just for you and has to be around in case you need it. Avoid calling Skittles® or other candies your "medicine" as this could really mess with a child's head. Be open and honest with kids, answer their questions and usually they will catch on quickly. When my kids used to ask for a glucose tablet, I'd say, "Are you low? Do you need to check your blood glucose?" Funny, they don't ask anymore.

A "rebound" blood glucose occurs when someone overtreats a low and ends up going high. For example, if someone's blood glucose level is 65 mg/dL and they treat with ½ cup orange juice and then follow that with some leftover pizza slices, a piece of cake with frosting, two cookies and some peanuts (basically anything that's not nailed down), they might end up in the 300s later on. It may be hard to believe, but experiencing hypoglycemia can actually make you want to eat this much (or more). Your brain might be telling you that you need only 4 oz. of juice, but it's also telling you to eat until you feel better. By the time your blood glucose is 300, you feel horrible all over again, and now it's from high blood glucose. This can turn into a vicious cycle.

If you are able to treat with 15 grams of carbohydrate and stop, that's great. If you do overtreat, however, do *NOT* beat yourself up over it. It's a very common phenomenon among people with diabetes. This tends to happen to me especially during those middle of the night lows. Fatigue makes it even harder to resist eating until the low feeling goes away. When this happens, you can take some insulin or go for a walk to offset the extra calories and prevent a high blood glucose later on. If you find yourself "chasing" blood glucose (overtreating a low, then going high, then taking insulin, then going low again, etc.) frequently, consider meeting with your health care provider to make some changes to your routine. A decrease in your insulin or other medication dose might be in order. It's never good to take more medication than you need, so if you notice that you are having frequent lows, make a change! This can especially happen if you have started exercising more or if you have lost weight. Nothing is more frustrating than getting all geared up, starting an exercise program, or other healthy lifestyle, and then being low all the time, having no energy, and being forced to consume all the calories you just burned off.

When your blood glucose is low, your energy level is low and so is your motivation level. It is physically challenging to treat a low blood glucose appropriately (i.e., stop eating after 15 grams of carb) or get anything done when your blood glucose is low. There are many reasons to talk to a professional about making changes to decrease the numbers of lows you experience. The downside to having frequent hypoglycemic events includes the following:

- Takes time out of your busy schedule
- Requires that you consume extra calories
- Puts you at risk for a fall, car accident, etc.
- Can affect relationships (can make you grumpy, spacy, or inconsistent)
- Decreases productivity (work, school)
- It's a hassle!

The downside to rebounding and going high later on includes

- Zaps your energy
- Can effect productivity
- Can affect relationships

- High blood glucose can contribute to long-term complications

One last thing about low blood glucose. Some people lose their symptoms of low blood glucose altogether. This is called "hypoglycemia unawareness," because these people are literally unaware when they are low. This is scary and dangerous, and people who experience this have some choices (imagine that). Continuous glucose monitoring (CGM), which was discussed in Chapter 6, is very helpful for people with hypoglycemia unawareness. CGM systems have alarms that alert people when their blood glucose level is dropping. These monitors also have "trending arrows" on the screen, which tell the user when and how fast their blood glucose level is dropping. Some people have hypoglycemia unawareness because they have kept their blood glucose levels very "tight" or close to normal for a while. These people can purposely run their blood glucose levels higher for a couple of weeks to improve or regain their low symptoms. Other people have hypoglycemia unawareness due to autonomic neuropathy. This is a diabetes-related complication that affects nerves that control involuntary actions in the body. In this case, continuous glucose monitoring is probably the safest approach.

Insulin pumps are a wonderful tool for intensively managing diabetes through fine-tuned insulin delivery. You can set "target ranges" for your blood glucose, and the pump (using programmed settings) will help you achieve these targets. It is common for people to experience much less hypoglycemia when using a pump rather than insulin injections. If you are currently using an insulin pump, but not taking advantage of these features, you might be pleasantly surprised. These are all things to discuss with your health care provider. At the very least, people with hypoglycemia unawareness need to be vigilant about checking blood glucose levels. The more you check, the more you know, and the more likely you are to catch a low.

A little exercise:

Make a plan for treating your lows. Decide what you will use to treat lows and then put low treatment items in places where you might need them (check off when you do it):

- ❒ car
- ❒ purse/backpack/beltpack/carry-on bag, etc.
- ❒ bedside table/bathroom
- ❒ with friend/family member
- ❒ school nurse/teachers/bus driver
- ❒ coach
- ❒ colleagues
- ❒ desk at work/school
- ❒ _____
- ❒ _____

Feeling confident that you are able to prevent, detect, and treat lows can lead you to have less fear of low blood glucose. In addition to being prepared for low blood glucose events and knowing how to handle them when they happen, be sure to talk to your health care provider about how to prevent them in the first place. Then you can get on with living your life!

Chapter 9
There's More To Diabetes Than Food

We don't let her have anything with sugar in it.
- family members of an 80-something woman with type 2 diabetes

People often mistakenly think food is all there is to diabetes: you get diabetes and you have to stop eating. Not exactly. There is a lot more to diabetes than food; in fact, everything relates to diabetes in some way. Without going into a huge scientific explanation, it's good to understand that diabetes is an endocrine disorder. Our endocrine system runs the long-term control of our bodies, such as growth, development and body temperature. Our nervous system is in charge of short-term control including muscles, reflexes and thoughts. The endocrine system runs on hormones, which are chemical messengers that are produced in one part of the body and then travel to other parts to do their jobs. Insulin is one of those hormones, and we cannot live without it. It's amazing how much work hormones do every minute of every day inside our bodies – and we aren't even aware of it! There are even some things going on in our bodies that no one understands yet.

When I stop and think about these things that I take for granted, it makes me honor and appreciate my body and what it does for me. It's also a nice reminder that I need to treat it well so it will keep doing those things. And food is just one part of the plan. It's about health and life. It's not just about diabetes. By understanding and addressing our whole being, we can be the healthiest and most whole person we were meant to be.

One Tuesday evening my neighbor called and asked if she could bring her son over. She wanted me to check his blood glucose because he'd been drinking a lot, urinating frequently, and not feeling good. I checked his blood glucose and the meter screen showed "ERROR: TOO HIGH TO READ." Somehow I got the words out and told them it was high. They ended up going to the Emergency Room that night and he was diagnosed with type 1 diabetes and admitted to the Intensive Care Unit. During the next three days my role went from helpful neighbor to diabetes educator (I'm the diabetes educator at our local hospital) to devastated neighbor-educator-person with type 1 diabetes. I could not figure out why this was hitting me so hard. I've spent my whole (diabetes) life proving that I'm fine. I can do anything. I can accomplish anything. I've never used diabetes as an excuse. I chose a career based on diabetes and often refer to my personal experiences or use my own experience with diabetes as an example. I have worked with many kids who have diabetes, several of whom were newly diagnosed. Why was this one having such a crushing effect on me when the others hadn't?

I sat at the hospital bedside and taught mom and son about insulin, the pancreas, high and low blood glucose, food, exercise, snacks – all the "survival skills." I prepared them for leaving our small hospital and "surviving" in the real world – or at least until they made their way to the nearest large diabetes center three hours away. But my emphasis during the time I sat there was on the fact that he was *no different*. I assured him that he was the *same kid* who could do the same things as he's always done. I realized afterward that I felt I had to prove to this 11-year-old that he was not broken or sick or in any way not whole.

It was through a conversation a few days later that I discovered the source of my struggle – why I had to do all this proving. I had never figured out my own diabetes "stuff" from years and years ago. I had never dealt with the fact that somewhere very deep down I questioned whether I was not whole or not perfect because of diabetes. I needed to *prove* that wasn't true. Keep in mind that I was diagnosed with type 1 diabetes during a time when parents and providers often did not assure kids that it was ok that this happened; that they weren't loved any less, or that they weren't a burden for requiring extra "work." But these are important things for a child (or adult) with a new diagnosis to hear.

The truth is, I have never really had to prove anything with my diabetes. Diabetes has never stopped me from doing or accomplishing anything. It has not negatively changed the course of my life and has in some ways positively changed it. I probably wouldn't have become a diabetes educator and I very likely wouldn't have written this book, had I not had diabetes. The truth is I'm *not* perfect. And I'm not perfect because I'm human, not because I have diabetes.

When people ask me questions about my diabetes, it's because they are confused, concerned or because they care – not because they are questioning *me*. Unfortunately, people with diabetes often feel judged (even if they are not). If someone without diabetes eats a candy bar, it's no big deal. If someone with diabetes takes some extra insulin and eats a candy bar, it's called "cheating." People with type 2 diabetes are often judged because they are overweight. Many people think the person with type 2 diabetes is at fault for getting it. Many people with type 2 feel this way about themselves.

Some of you may relate to this, some may not. The point is that *you are not to blame for your diabetes*. Having diabetes does not make you a bad person – even if you make unhealthy food choices at times! That just makes you a normal person. No one deserves to have diabetes, and some people get it anyway. For those of you who love someone with diabetes: treat them as the same person they were before they were diagnosed. Avoid nagging, complaining, blaming, or judging them. If you have concerns about their eating habits, approach it as just that – a concern. As difficult as it may be to accept, your loved one is in charge - or will be when they are old enough - of managing their own diabetes. As you know, this book is about choices. What we eat, what we do, and how we live are choices. You can choose to support them, encourage them and love them. And that will lead to much better outcomes than blaming and nagging.

Stress and Diabetes

Stress is the body's way of responding to a demand - whether that is perceived as a good or bad thing. Stress can be emotional – getting in a fight, a death in the family, a new job or a move. Stress can be physical – infection, illness, or pain. Stress can be hormonal – PMS, menopause, pregnancy, or taking medications that are hormones or steroids (cortisone injections, for example). And the natural stress response involves a rise in blood glucose. Stress triggers the release of certain hormones in the human body. These hormones tell the body to make glucose and send it into the bloodstream. I like to use the example of meeting a bear on your path. This would be stressful! The fight or flight response kicks in and your body knows that the last thing you need to think about is eating, so it graciously provides glucose for you. Those who are able to make insulin can counteract that glucose and use it productively. But for those of us with diabetes, this whole scenario just makes our blood glucose level high.

Stress can be acute, for instance, a death in the family or an accident or injury. That type of stress typically does a number on blood glucose levels. Stress can also be chronic, for instance, working in a job you hate day in and day out. Chronic stress tends to lead to overeating and neglecting diabetes self-care tasks like checking blood glucose or taking medications or exercising. As you can imagine, this is just a vicious cycle, which is why stress management is an important part of diabetes management. Managing stress may involve developing or adopting coping mechanisms for when stress occurs, or it may mean thinking about other options to alleviate the stress. If your job is the source of stress, perhaps it's time for a new job or career. If the people you hang out with cause you stress, you may need to talk to them about it or find new friends. Perhaps you could try medication (work with a health care professional), counseling, or something else. It is important to use or develop your skills for coping with stress. You may already have mechanisms in place, such as meditation, prayer, yoga, support groups, the Diabetes Online Community, diabetes camp, or volunteer work. If you are already using one or more of these activities, continue to do so, and if not, consider starting.

Some people believe that stress actually brought on their diabetes. If you experienced an extremely stressful event or period in your life just prior to being diagnosed with diabetes, there is a chance that stress was a trigger. However, you were most likely already set up for getting diabetes genetically, physically, or otherwise, and the stress may have just sped up the process a little.

A little exercise:

Write down the things in your life that are causing you stress:

_____

_____

_____

_____

_____

_____

Write down some ways you can cope with stress (hints: listen to music, call a friend, go for a walk):

_____

_____

_____

_____

_____

You could even write these ideas on little pieces of paper and put them in a jar. Next time you are really stressed out, pull one of them out of the jar and do what it says! As you can imagine, attitude plays a role in managing stress. We can get bogged down in negative thoughts, or we can own our situation and make it better - whatever that takes. At the very least we can have a positive attitude and find something to be grateful for or happy about each day.

Food Anxiety

There is a phenomenon I have observed in people with diabetes, and I like to call it *food anxiety*. Food anxiety tends to occur when people with diabetes find themselves outside of their comfort zone. This is a situation where they are not in control of food for any number of reasons, and the following are a few examples:

- Someone (perhaps a parent or spouse) is hovering over them and questioning everything they put in their mouths.

178

- They are staying in another person's home, a hotel, a conference center, and don't have easy access to food.
- They are on a "campus" where food is available only at certain times of the day.

I've seen (and I've experienced personally) people run out to the nearest convenience store or fast food restaurant to load up on food when they feel food anxiety. They may hide food in their room or suitcase. All this does is lead to a feeling of doing something wrong. It's ok to keep food with you, in the event that you need or want something to eat and it's not otherwise available. Sometimes the tendency is to want unhealthy items during those situations. I have seen adolescents rebel when their parents watch or question everything they do. They might literally be "closet eaters," or they might snack in other secret places. I've seen cars full of candy and fast food wrappers. I have memories of being with a group of camp counselors and heading for the local donut shop or convenience store as soon as we had some time off. The food in the dining hall wasn't horrible, but we felt we couldn't eat what and when we wanted, so this is how we responded. Open communication about food might lead to less secretive eating and maybe even healthier choices.

Food Scrutiny and the Food Police

It isn't possible to write a book about diabetes and food and *not* have a section on *The Food Police*. People with diabetes are plagued with being watched and sometimes just worrying about being watched when food is involved. I call this *food scrutiny*. The food police are those people who comment about, question, critique (judge), or scrutinize what people with diabetes put on their plates and in their mouths. I would guess that every person with diabetes has, at some point, dealt with the food police. I could fill an entire chapter with my encounters with the force, but I will just give a few here.

- At a family reunion I went to the food table and filled my plate. As I was walking back to sit down, an aunt leaned over my plate and said, "Let me see what you took." She was not kidding! I had to stop and show her my plate. She commented on each item and then said something like, "Oh, you took a cookie…"

- After giving birth to my first child, I was looking forward to the fancy dinner they give every new mom: steak or salmon, potato, veggies, and a piece of cheesecake for dessert. When my tray arrived the nurse informed me that the person in dietary was refusing to give me the cheesecake because I have diabetes. I said, "Get her on the phone" – and I wasn't kidding! I talked to the woman in dietary and I got my cheesecake.

- When I was a kid my mother took my siblings and me to a museum-type place with another family. When we were just about finished, the kids were asking for ice cream and the other mother said, "No one is having ice cream because Jane can't." Talk about winning friends!

- Then there's the passive food police stunt where the person is showing you the spread and says something like, "I'm not sure if we have anything you can eat."

Sometimes people mistake *me* for the food police. I live in a small town, and I am constantly bumping into patients in public places. I once saw a patient in the grocery store and she was eating something (I hadn't even noticed). She pointed it out and said, "I'm busted – I'm eating chocolate."

Sometimes the tables are turned and we actually do become the food police. I often hear comments from patients in the hospital such as, "I can't believe the breakfast they served me – it was all carbohydrates! I would never eat that at home!" I am guilty of being the food police at conferences or meetings where they serve high-calorie foods and sugared soda to drink. I often wish they would serve healthy options (fresh fruit and vegetables, whole grains) and a variety of drinks, including some that don't have sugar. More and more are doing this, which is great to see (and eat).

There are also blood glucose police out there: people who are really anxious to see you check your blood glucose and then have all sorts of comments about the result. I sometimes don't mind explaining, and other times I really don't want to check in front of anyone because I'm not up for it. Just like the food police, these people are generally not trying to be mean or judgmental. For the most part, they care about us or are genuinely curious or concerned. Many people who don't have diabetes are not well-informed about the disease and its management. They may know only that Great Aunt Whoever died from diabetes-related complications and they don't want that to happen to you. Back in the day (prior to the early 1990s) the health care community really did ban sugar and this is what the general public remembers, so we have to cut them some slack and keep working to inform the masses about what we know now about diabetes.

Language

You may notice that I don't use the word "diabetic" anywhere in this book. In fact, if you see that word, it is part of a direct quote or a typo!! I don't use the word "diabetic" because it is a label. I feel that calling a person by their disease mistakenly leads to *defining* a person as their disease, or making it the focus of the person. You are learning how important I think attitude is, so you can imagine that defining oneself as their disease would not equal a healthy attitude.

We are so much more than diabetes! We are people, friends, moms, dads, sons, daughters, professionals, students, hard workers, slackers, athletes – whatever! – who *happen* to have diabetes. I have a friend from diabetes camp who coined the term, "the 'ic' word." How appropriate! I've always loved that, because if you think about it… "ick." I also don't use "diet" whenever possible, because it has become such a negatively charged word. People with diabetes are not on a "diet," they are making choices. If I really needed to use the word "diet" in this book, you will notice that I have put it in quotation marks. Another "four-letter-word" for people with diabetes is "cheat." I will spare you a long, drawn-out sermon by saying that people with (or without) diabetes are not "cheating" when they eat certain foods or drink certain beverages. They are simply making a choice. Amen.

There are other words I steer clear of when talking/writing about diabetes: "good," "bad," "test," "compliant," "non-compliant," "should," "shouldn't," and "control" to name a few. When I talk to family members of kids with diabetes I mention the damage these words can do. Kids often feel that *they* are bad if someone says their numbers are bad. Adults often feel this way too. No one would ever feel bad about a blood glucose reading if somewhere along the line someone hadn't told them it was bad. I can't tell you how often I hear people say, "I'm bad" or "I've been bad" or even worse – "I'm a bad diabetic." You say that enough, and you might convince yourself – *then* what are your chances of success?

I once had a camper (teen-aged girl) who wouldn't come out of the cabin to tell me her blood glucose level (we were doing breakfast insulin). It turned out that she was in the 200s and she truly believed that 1) she was a bad person and 2) I or someone else would be upset with her for having a blood glucose at that level. What a way to feel! It's just a number. A number that gives us the information to guide the next decision in our daily diabetes management: more insulin? More food? More exercise? Do nothing?

I don't use "test" to describe blood glucose monitoring because it's not a test. There's no grade, evaluation, pass or fail. I usually say "check" because I'm checking to see what my blood glucose is doing. It's just information and it is just for the person with diabetes. Some of you might be thinking, "But it's also for the physician (nurse practitioner, PA, etc.)" and I would respond that while yes, health care providers may – hopefully – take a look at the numbers, and while they may make suggestions or recommendations for adjustments based on these numbers, the ultimate responsibility for making choices based on the numbers always goes back to the person with diabetes.

And that brings me to "compliance." Compliance means meeting someone else's expectations. While health care providers teach, guide and serve as a resource, the expectation really comes from inside *us*. We do the work and we reap the rewards. We comply with state or federal agencies, but when it comes to our health, it's all about choices. Your health is truly yours and it is up to you to achieve it and maintain it. If you set health goals for yourself, it is up to you to meet them. Historically, our health care system was not designed to support this philosophy. As a result, we often feel that we are not in charge of our health. But we are. In the case of a chronic condition like diabetes, we especially are. No one is going to come home with us and make sure we poke our finger, take our medication, or dish up a certain amount of food. Each person with diabetes is the central player on their health care team. Physicians, nurses, dietitians, educators, physical therapists, social workers, counselors, exercise physiologists, pharmacists, etc., are members of the team. They each contribute in unique ways, but the person with diabetes is in charge. The person with diabetes has *100%* of the responsibility for their condition, for the choices they make in managing it, and, in turn, for their successes!

> **Tasty Morsel (of information):** There are many people who have diabetes and cannot care for themselves. Young children, elderly people and people with special needs or disabilities may require caregivers to check their blood glucose, administer medications, or even prepare food and feed them. These people may not have 100% of the responsibility for their diabetes.

Just as I am not the Food Police, I am certainly not the "Language Police." If people want to call themselves "diabetics" that is their choice. For the reasons I've just explained, I only ask that you don't refer to others (or me) using these terms. I have experienced and observed that our language shapes our responses in life. Language can build us up and help us feel strong and empowered. It can also tear us down and make us feel small and incompetent. Or at fault. Or a victim. I truly believe that using strength-based language, and surrounding ourselves with people who do the same can lead us to a more positive attitude and therefore better outcomes. I am learning more about this every day. I realize there are still some words I use that can be replaced, and it's an ongoing process. The point is to be open to changing how I look at things and what I say.

Special Circumstances Worth Mentioning

Life throws challenges at us constantly. Some are easier to handle than others. Two that deserve further discussion include pregnancy and terminal illness. These two situations have come up frequently in my professional life. Both can be a challenge when managing diabetes.

Pregnancy

I've managed diabetes through pregnancy twice, and it was a lot of work. The first time I was militaristic about eating times, types of food, and amounts. My poor husband could tell you that every time we tried to eat out I insisted on eating only at certain places (or rather, insisting on *not* eating at certain places). The second time, knowing that it all worked out ok, and having a baby to take care of already, I wasn't quite as crazy about the food thing, but I still paid close attention.

Women who have diabetes (and their babies) benefit *greatly* from taking pregnancy very seriously and planning for it. Being pregnant with diabetes is doable – and it takes a lot of work. If you are planning to get pregnant, know that going in! I assure you (from personal experience) that the end results – healthy baby and healthy mom – are well worth the effort. Women with diabetes who keep their hemoglobin A1C in a safe range, lower their chances of problems to about the same as those without diabetes.

Pregnant women with pre-existing diabetes need to monitor blood glucose levels frequently (before and after meals, etc.), bring down or "correct" high blood glucose as soon as possible, be prepared for and treat low blood glucose, and check urine for ketones. They also have frequent visits to the obstetrician, endocrinologist or primary care provider, ophthalmologist (eye doctor) and maybe others. If she is living in a remote area (like I was during pregnancy), she will benefit from going to a large hospital/clinic for a fetal echocardiogram. This is a precaution to make sure the baby's heart is healthy. If there are any problems, the woman may want to deliver in a bigger hospital with specialists who can care for the baby right away at birth. As mentioned earlier, a wonderful resource for women with diabetes who are pregnant or thinking about becoming pregnant is Kathryn Palmer's book, *When You're a Parent with Diabetes*.

Exercise is an important part of managing diabetes before, during and after pregnancy, and eating well is key. Cravings are an interesting challenge: I craved high-fat foods like Fritos® and certain items from McDonald's. Those not only make my blood glucose high when I'm eating them, but thanks to the fat content they stay with me (keep my blood glucose high) for several hours. How nice would it be to crave salads and fruit? Oh well. It's ok to give in to cravings (in moderation, if possible) – and then try to take insulin or go for a walk to balance the blood glucose level and keep it in a safe range.

Morning sickness is another challenge for pregnant women with diabetes. Just as with any sickness, the recommendation is that you check your blood glucose more frequently and take in whatever food/beverages you can. Sip on some regular ginger ale or eat some broth or crackers. Knowing where your blood glucose level is will help with dosing insulin.

For women who take insulin during pregnancy, the amounts that are required can be pretty overwhelming. I was appalled at how much insulin I needed during the second and third trimesters (it's common to run low and require less insulin during the first trimester). I had a mantra that I repeated over and over to myself: "Insulin is my friend." Insulin requirements can double, if not triple during pregnancy! Someone with pre-existing type 2 diabetes, who managed with "diet" and exercise or pills prior to becoming pregnant, will likely require insulin during pregnancy.

Women with gestational diabetes mellitus (GDM) (diabetes that is diagnosed during pregnancy – usually in the second half) don't have diabetes when they get pregnant, so planning is not possible. In this case, it's important to start checking blood glucose levels, eating healthy, well-balanced meals, and exercising as soon as they are diagnosed. For women with GDM, medication may or may not be necessary. Women who had GDM during a pregnancy have an increased risk of getting diabetes later in life. As always, it is important to keep up the healthy habits you started during pregnancy. Talk to your health care provider about when and how often to get screened for diabetes after you deliver your baby.

Terminal Illness and Diabetes

Despite the fact that when I was a kid I truly believed that you can get only one major health issue, people with diabetes sometimes get cancer and people with cancer sometimes get diabetes too. It sounds like a cruel trick, but it can happen for a variety of reasons:

- Some cancer medications cause elevated blood glucose levels.

- The cancer itself can affect the body's ability to function properly.
- Weight gain during cancer treatment can bring on diabetes.
- Some people were going to get diabetes anyway and the timing was just really *bad.*

Regardless of the person's prognosis, diabetes is not necessarily the priority during cancer treatment. If high blood glucose levels are causing him/her to feel lethargic and contributing to depression and/or generally feeling sick, it is helpful to find a medication that will bring the blood glucose level down to a safe and healthy range. It is possible, then, to eat what tastes and feels good. For someone whose cancer is terminal, feeling in control of *something* is important and for some, it is food. If the cancer is treatable, focusing on healthy choices (that taste good) and exercise is beneficial to providing energy and strength during treatment. Healthy eating and exercise habits can also lead to better health after cancer.

Diabetes and Depression

Depression occurs in 8 to 27% of people with diabetes (20). It is twice as common for people with diabetes to experience depression as it is for the general population. Believe it or not, depression can also lead to diabetes, and those who are experts in this area aren't clear on which comes first. Diabetes and depression are a challenging combination because depression can lead to not taking medications; not checking blood glucose levels; not exercising; missing appointments; worsening blood glucose levels; and higher risk of foot ulcers. Here is a list of some of the signs and symptoms of depression:

- Overwhelming feelings of sadness or unhappiness

- Irritability or frustration
- Loss of interest or pleasure in normal activities
- Reduced sex drive
- Inability to sleep or excessive sleeping
- Changes in appetite – decreased or increased appetite leading to weight loss or weight gain
- Agitation or restlessness
- Slowed thinking
- Indecisiveness, decreased concentration
- Fatigue and loss of energy
- Feeling of worthlessness
- Crying for no apparent reason
- Unexplained pain or headaches
- Frequent thoughts of death, dying, or suicide

Depression zaps motivation, and diabetes management calls for a pretty big dose of motivation. If you suspect that you or someone you care about is experiencing depression, please contact your health care provider to ask about effective resources. Fortunately, depression can be managed with therapy/counseling, medications, or other approaches.

Diabetes Distress

There is also a phenomenon that has been named *diabetes distress*, which occurs in many people, but is different from clinical depression. Diabetes distress is characterized by a sense of burden or feeling overwhelmed by the tasks and responsibilities of daily diabetes management. It challenges emotional and physical well-being and can lead to poor health outcomes. Setting small, attainable goals is one way to manage diabetes distress. There is a screening tool available to determine if you have diabetes distress. If you are interested in learning more, talk to your health care provider.

Diabetes and the Elderly

I have a policy when I am at work at the hospital. I typically get a referral on every patient who comes in and happens to have diabetes. It doesn't matter what they are in the hospital for – typically it's not diabetes. Because I live in a ski town, we see a lot of patients who have fractured limbs or knee injuries, and we also see a lot of patients with joint replacements. When I get a consult on a patient who is 80 years or older, I go into the room, say hi, introduce myself and ask if there is anything I can do for them in terms of their diabetes. I do not try to ram information or recommendations down their throats (hopefully I don't do that with younger patients either). I once heard that people who are diagnosed with diabetes at age 70 or older are not going to die from diabetes complications. I also believe that people who have had diabetes for a while and are in their 80s or 90s are not going to suddenly develop complications like eye or kidney disease (unless they are already coming on).

I believe that if someone has lived into their 80s or 90s, they have obviously done something right! They deserve to continue doing what they are doing and enjoy as much quality of life as possible for as long as they are here on earth. Many elderly people do not have the appetite that they had when they were younger. The concern may be more with their getting enough to eat rather than restricting their calories or intake. Some elderly diabetes patients manage their blood glucose very intensively, and sometimes for safety reasons I recommend that they ease up a bit and run their numbers slightly higher (for example, target 140 to 180 mg/dL instead of 100 mg/dL). I also focus on giving elderly people as much independence as possible. I personally dread the thought of having someone else give me my injections or check my blood glucose for me. As long as it is possible, I want to be involved (ok, in charge) of my own diabetes management. So for all the family members, like the ones quoted at the beginning of the chapter, who are serving as food police for their elderly parents, please consider backing off and giving Mom or Dad some control. Let them eat what they enjoy. The important thing is that they are safe and feel good, which equates to blood glucose levels that are not too high or too low. Instead of restricting them, talk to the health care professional about a safe and healthy blood glucose target range for your loved one.

Chapter 10
No Wrong Answers

I've started doing crafts to get my hands off cigarettes and food
60-something woman with type 2 diabetes

This is a conversation that, for some people, might be more productive in a live setting than in a book, but let's have it anyway. Diabetes can be frustrating, overwhelming, or just a plain-old pain in the butt. It's very important to figure out where your head is. If you find that you are buried in negative thoughts, it's time to fix that. I won't try to tell you that diabetes is fun or exciting, but we definitely can be positive about it. A positive attitude toward diabetes helps keep your head clear, which helps you focus and get things done. You have a much higher chance of success both in the short- and long-term, if you stay positive.

Often it helps to figure out what motivates you in order to get up, get out and take on diabetes. If we are committed to doing something, we can do it. If you figure out why you want to be here and what you want to accomplish, then you can manage your diabetes, live a healthy life and accomplish what you set out to do.

Some people are motivated by family: they want to know their grandchildren, or attend someone's graduation or wedding. Others are motivated by success at work, school, hobbies, sports, or volunteer work. What motivates you to take care of yourself? Do you have children? Grandchildren? Do you have career goals? Is there something you want to accomplish or achieve in your lifetime – or sooner?

Think about all the incredibly successful people who are out there living with diabetes and enjoying what they love to do: athletes, musicians, actors, and others. In addition to the famous types, there are people with diabetes who work in all sorts of professions. You can do whatever you set your mind to do.

Whatever gets you energized and excited can be what motivates you to take care of yourself. With diabetes we take care of ourselves by doing the daily tasks involved with managing the disease. If your blood glucose is in order, you can be more productive in the activities that make up your life. Not to mention managing your diabetes *now* can lead to your being around (and in a healthier state) to enjoy those things that you look forward to.

> **Tasty Morsel (of information):** If you do not enjoy the activities in your life (your job, the people you hang out with, your hobbies), then find some new ones, for goodness sake! This is it! You've got one life to live, so own it: do what you enjoy whenever possible. Take a good look at yourself, your life, and what you are doing. Does it make sense? Does it bring you satisfaction, fulfillment, and/or enjoyment? If so, carry on. If not, it's time to figure some things out. Talk to someone, read some books, go online, whatever it takes to find what clicks for you. What makes you excited and brings out the positive attitude in you? Remember that motivation is all about what matters to *you* and not anyone else. If you are doing this for someone else, you are less likely to succeed.

There is a little activity you can try on your own that can help you figure out what motivates you. It involves answering some questions: Why do you want to manage your diabetes daily? And why is that important? And why is that important? And why is that important? And why is that important?

Known as the "5 Whys," this approach was originally developed (for use by Toyota) to determine the root cause of a problem. It has been adapted over time, and used in a variety of settings and scenarios. For our purposes, it helps us get to the root of what motivates us to make a change. Figuring this out can even jumpstart our ***attitude***. Here's an example:

1. Why do you want to manage your diabetes daily?
   So my blood glucose levels will be in a healthy range.
2. And why is that important?
   Because I think more clearly when my blood glucose is consistently in a healthy range.
3. And why is that important?
   So I can get/stay organized and be more productive and efficient.
4. And why is that important?
   Because I want to stop feeling like I am going in circles.
5. And why is that important?
   Because then I will have more quality time and quality relationships with family and friends.

If you cut out the middle stuff, you end up with *It's important for me to manage my diabetes daily so that I will have more quality time and quality relationships with family and friends.* And you can use this little exercise to find out about other areas of your life too – relationships, career choices, and so on. ***Try it yourself!!***

A little exercise:

Why do you want to (fill in your goal)

_____

_____

_____

And why is that important?

_____

_____

_____

And why is that important?

_____

_____

_____

And why is that important?

_____

_____

_____

And why is that important?

_____

_____

_____

Another motivational activity you can do is to create a poster (or 8.5 x 11 paper or sticky note or an album) with messages and pictures that represent your goal(s). Hang it where you'll see it regularly – or carry it with you – and it will remind you to stay motivated. These are *your* goals - not someone's else's; therefore, they are meaningful to you. When you are ready to start setting goals, there are some important points to keep in mind:

- Set yourself up for success, not failure, by setting realistic, doable, achievable goals.
- Make your goals measurable (so you can determine when you've met them) and break them down into small chunks.

- Give yourself deadlines/set dates for achieving your goals.
- Write down your goals and look at them often.
- Cross them out as you achieve them.

Some people refer to these as SMART goals, which stands for Specific, Measurable, Attainable, Realistic and Timely. Think of what you want to change or take on in your life; think about why you want to do it; go do it! It's important not to make goal-setting and goal-achievement sound too simple. Many of our goals are very difficult to achieve, and we need to acknowledge that the road to success may not be easy or fun. Being realistic but not negative can help us stay focused as well as, if not more than (in some cases) being positive. Heidi Grant Halvorson has written an excellent book about goal-setting. It is based on research and it's called *Succeed: How We Can Reach Our Goals*.

A little exercise:

Write down your goals. Don't forget to make them measurable and give them deadlines (dates).

My list of goals:

_____

_____

_____

_____

_____

_____

_____

_____

_____

Breaking the Cycle (in order to break the habit)

If you are trying to make healthier eating choices, but you keep going to places that serve unhealthy food, it's going to be quite challenging to make a change. I was eating lunch at one of those 50's diner-type places right after meeting with a patient. The patient had heart disease, high blood pressure, high cholesterol, and high blood glucose. I was sitting in this restaurant, surrounded by burgers, bacon, French fries, and milk shakes, and could not help thinking about this patient and others just like her. So many people were raised on these foods and consider them "comfort" foods. Going out for a meal was special, and why shouldn't we enjoy ourselves with big, huge helpings? That's what is served, and we paid for it, after all. I ask every new patient, "How many times do you eat out in a typical week?" and they often forget about lunch. Eating lunch out (and for many, breakfast too) can become part of the routine. When we eat out, we usually don't know how much we're getting or how it was prepared. There are many extra calories (often "hidden") in restaurant food. Portions are typically very large. If we stick with eating comfort foods occasionally (like once or twice a month), we'll have a much easier time achieving our health goals.

Another way to break the cycle is to get help. If it helps to talk to someone – do it! Contact your local diabetes educator, a therapist/counselor, a clergy person, a friend or relative. Tell someone what you are trying to do and ask for their support, cheerleading, and listening ear; whatever it is that you need. Use your resources. There are countless resources available for people with diabetes – use them. The World Wide Web is a wonderful source of information/support for people with diabetes. There are diabetes "social networks" and informational websites. You can look up the carbohydrate content of any food online; you can find an "e-mail pal" to compare notes, swap stories, etc. The Diabetes Online Community (DOC) is a network of people who write about their diabetes experiences on "blogs." I have purposely avoided making a list of these blogs because it would undoubtedly be outdated as soon as the book is published. There are more popping up every day! An internet search for "diabetes social networks" or "diabetes blogs" will yield plenty. Your local community likely has several resources for helping you with weight loss, exercise, support and much more. Perhaps you could join a book club or get back into a craft you once enjoyed to take your mind off of diabetes for a while.

If you are trying to quit smoking, you may have an easier time if you stop going to the same places where you have always smoked. You may find it's better to stop spending time with people who smoke. If you want to start making healthier eating choices, you may need to cut down or cut out visits to some types of eating establishments. And when you do find yourself back in one of those places, work hard to make the healthiest choices possible: remember to skip or share it, have a salad (with a healthy dressing), or take a walk afterward.

Sometimes it takes a little effort to find a "healthy" place to eat, but in general, things are coming around. Fast food chains have added some healthier items, and restaurants with healthier themes are popping up all over. Even convenience stores are carrying healthier snacks such as fruit and nuts. Just like the former smoker, who knows what situations they have to avoid in order not to have a cigarette, you will learn where to go for a healthier meal – and which places to avoid. Hope Warshaw has written two helpful books about eating out: *Eat Out, Eat Right: The Guide to Healthier Eating Out* and *Guide to Healthy Restaurant Eating*.

Breaking habits is often about distraction. The quote at the beginning of the chapter is from a woman who worked hard to quit smoking and stop snacking between meals. She was trying to improve her health in two ways: by cutting out cigarettes and managing her blood glucose. By taking up crafts, she found that she could keep herself busy (distracted) and therefore didn't think about smoking or eating as much.

> **Tasty Morsel (of information):** Smoking/chewing tobacco is deadly for everyone, and even more so for those with diabetes. All the scary things that diabetes puts you at risk for, are also risks from smoking. The problem with combining diabetes and smoking is the risk multiplies, not two times, but hundreds of times. If you have diabetes and you smoke, do whatever it takes to quit smoking. You can use the tools in this book to help yourself live a healthy life without tobacco. You deserve it!

Barriers

Barriers are the hurdles we have to navigate to achieve our goals. Barriers (just like goals) are different for different people. Some barriers to quitting smoking include living with someone who smokes, or having a social life that revolves around smoking – and you can probably think of barriers to making healthy food choices too. If you are serious about achieving your goals, though, the first step is coming to terms with your barriers. And then figuring out how to get past them. For instance, if snacking at work is a barrier (many workplaces have all sorts of unhealthy foods laying around that are hard to avoid), perhaps bringing in your own healthy snacks is a way to overcome that barrier. Perhaps you can talk yourself out of eating the unhealthy snacks. Maybe you could carry your goals in your pocket/purse and pull them out every time you are confronted with unhealthy snacks, as a quick reminder to stay motivated. You might even consider talking to your colleagues and/or supervisor about either 1) discontinuing the snacks, 2) moving them to a less prominent location, or 3) bringing more healthy snacks such as fruit or veggies. You might be surprised at how many co-workers would thank you for making the suggestion.

A little exercise:

Make a list of your barriers to healthy choices and ideas for what you can do to overcome them:

Barriers   Ways to overcome them

_____   _____

_____   _____

_____   _____

_____   _____

_____   _____

Guilt is Ineffective

With diabetes comes a lot of guilt. Even the most well-intentioned health care providers have slipped in words that can make patients feel guilty. Like the term "compliance," there are only a few instances where guilt is warranted. If you steal something from another person, it would be appropriate to feel guilty. If you cheat on a math test or plagiarize a paper, guilt is in order, but if your blood glucose is high, or if you eat an extra "treat," you don't need to feel guilty. As I mentioned earlier, I think the words we use when discussing diabetes really do matter, because they can have a tendency to contribute to guilt. For instance, if someone is told they are "cheating" when they eat an extra snack, why wouldn't they feel guilty? They have been made to feel they've done something wrong. If someone gets a "bad" number on their "test," guilt is a normal response (they didn't study hard enough or perform well enough).

Guilt is a useless behavior was once our mantra at diabetes camp. Guilt goes with something that belongs to someone else, not ourselves. When we manage our own diabetes we make our own choices. If we make a choice that we regret, we can do it differently next time. We can learn from our mistakes. Sometimes we make choices that may not be the healthiest (like eating a candy bar), but we make them consciously, and we enjoy the taste or experience. We can take a walk or take a little insulin if our blood glucose is high. We have not committed a crime, we are not bad people and we are not guilty.

It may seem like I'm oversimplifying the guilt thing. I know that at one time I felt guilty when I ate something that made my blood glucose high. In fact, I felt guilty when I saw a high number on my meter. As many people have, I went through phases where I would avoid checking my blood glucose if I thought it was elevated – I just didn't want to see a high number and then experience that awful feeling. Over the years I have become able to see those numbers for what they are – numbers and nothing more. They don't scare or intimidate me, or make me feel guilty. Sometimes I add a little commentary when I see a particular number: "bummer" or "nice" or "woops" or "huh"? No matter how you slice it, the number provides information that I can use to make a decision. It does not make me good or bad, guilty or innocent. Approaching blood glucose levels this way has helped me stay positive and balanced and focused.

One thing that helps me when I see a high number on my meter is to figure out why. I approach it like a science project. If I know exactly why my blood glucose is elevated, I can do something different next time. Earlier I mentioned that sometimes blood glucose readings make no sense, and so there are definitely times when I just have to shrug, get over it and move on. Overall I spend less time with elevated blood glucose levels not only because I'm not afraid to see them when they happen, but because I do something about them quickly and get them right back down to a "happy" level.

> **Tasty Morsel (of information)**: Sometimes I think type 1 diabetes is easier to manage than type 2 because if my blood glucose level is high I can take insulin to "correct" it. People with type 2 diabetes often don't manage with insulin, and there can be a tendency to just run high. However, if you have type 2 diabetes and you see a high reading, you can go for a walk, talk to your provider about increasing your medication (if you take any), or make different choices with your food. And all of us, regardless of diabetes type, can choose to have a positive attitude!

Visualization

Another suggestion for how you might overcome barriers is visualization. This is something you can do – wherever you are – to help you focus on positive outcomes. You can visualize part of your body (in good health) or yourself having achieved a goal (however that looks to you) or something else completely. I have been visualizing healthy eyes for over ten years. I credit Catherine Feste (she wrote *365 Daily Meditations for Diabetes*, check it out!) and Lee Pulos (*The Power of Visualization* – a very helpful tool) with helping me figure out how to use visualization. Visualization is calming, empowering, and can be beneficial to your health. It is well-known that athletes use visualization to improve their performance, and this is yet another way it can help give positive results. Meditation and prayer are closely related to visualization and can be used instead of, or in combination with visualization.

Simple steps to visualization:

1. Choose a routine time to do your visualizing; preferably a time when you have quiet and solitude. (I visualize at night before I go to bed.)

2. Create a mental image of your goal and the steps it will take to reach it. (My image is healthy eyes. If you need help with the image, get a copy of a photo. I obtained a photo of a healthy retina, which is the back of the eye.)

3. Come up with a mantra and write it down. It's ok to more than one mantra. (My mantra for my eyes goes like this: *My eyes are perfectly healthy; my eyes are healed and clear. My optic discs are bright, the central point for supple, healthy vessels. My optic nerves and muscles are strong and functioning perfectly. My maculas are clear and normal. My retinas are healthy and clear.*)

4. Look at your image/list of steps (either in your mind or on paper) and say your mantra. (Eventually you will have it memorized.)

A little exercise:

Write down your goal/image

_____

Write down your mantra

_____

_____

_____

A very important point to remember about visualization is that you still have to do the work to make it happen. Athletes visualize winning a competition, but they still work out and train for the event. Likewise, we still check blood glucose levels, take medications, make healthy food choices and exercise. In her book, *Succeed: How We Can Reach Our Goals*, Heidi Grant Halvorson explains that it's not enough to just visualize the outcome you're after. We also need to visualize doing the steps it will take to achieve that outcome, which can help us to actually take those steps.

Internal vs. External

Some people have a tendency to be internally regulated, while others are more externally regulated. Internal regulation means that you respond to "internal" cues from your body – how you feel, how your clothes fit, your energy level, etc. Externally regulated people tend to respond to outside "controls" like calorie-counting and weigh-ins. There can also be a happy medium between the two for those who are somewhere in the middle.

Take a moment to think about which types of cues you respond better to. How does this show up in your life? Are you a numbers person? Do you need to see the scale every morning or weekly? Or do you know how you are doing based on the way you feel, or how your clothes fit? Do you need someone else to tell you you're doing a good job, or to acknowledge your success? Or would you prefer to keep to yourself? Or are you somewhere in between?

If you are internally regulated, you may not want to join a weight loss program. Perhaps reading, discussing with "friends" on the internet, or setting personal goals would work more effectively for you. Internal cues include recognizing hunger and fullness. Many people lose the ability to feel hungry and full. This can be a very effective technique for those who are internally regulated. Listen to your body – is it telling you

you are hungry? It's important to eat when you are hungry, in order to avoid overeating later on. When you eat, listen to your body's cues indicating when you are full – it really will tell you. Slowing down at meal time helps too. If you eat too fast, you might just miss the full cues and eat right through them. If you have not been in touch with your body's hunger and fullness cues in a while (or ever), it can take some time and focus to learn them. Stick with it, though, because when it happens it's pretty rewarding. A good resource on this topic is the book *Intuitive Eating* by Evelyn Tribole and Elyse Resch.

If you are externally regulated, a weight loss program might be a better choice for you. You might respond better to something that gives you outside accountability, such as showing up to meetings and weigh-ins, counting your calories (carbs), and filling out reports or journals. Joining a gym and exercising with other people who count on you to show up might be effective (find another friend who is also externally regulated).

Using techniques that address the opposite of your preferences can actually backfire. For instance, if someone who prefers internal regulation tries to use measuring cups and scales in the kitchen, or gets on the scale daily, they might get extremely discouraged and throw in the towel. I've already mentioned what has happened when I've joined gyms in the past. I have not gone to the gym and I've wasted money on the membership. I am content to do my walking on a treadmill in my garage and I rarely skip doing it. This does not mean that I am internally regulated in all areas, but I do tend to lean that way. On the other hand, someone who responds to external cues, and tries to "just do it on their own," may get discouraged with a lack of success, in which case a gym membership, or at least having the support of a walking partner, might be a better choice.

Recording blood glucose readings is another example of where internal vs. external regulation would play a role. If you are externally regulated, you might be more likely to either write down every blood glucose reading in a logbook or take advantage of software that allows you to download your readings and create tables, graphs, and such. The more internal types might just leave the information inside the meter and let the health care provider download it at each visit. Or they may forget to bring their meter to visits.

Perhaps you are externally regulated and by nature you need to talk more about your diabetes. This might help some people keep it a priority or focus. As long as diabetes does not take over your life and overshadow important things like who you are or your interests and activities, this is fine. On the other hand, some who are internally regulated might take it as far as not telling anyone about their diabetes. This could be dangerous if they needed help, for instance, with a low blood glucose. The bottom line is to be aware of how you are wired – what cues guide you most effectively – and use that information to benefit you in managing your diabetes and staying healthy.

Importance vs. Confidence

Another way to look at motivation is to figure out what is important to you (checking blood glucose levels, taking medication(s), exercising, watching portions, eating vegetables, etc.) and then determining how confident you are that you can accomplish each of those activities. If you are not confident, why is that? If you can identify what keeps you from being confident, you can start to consider ways to solve the problem, make a change, or whatever it will take. You might find out that you need to work on just one thing at a time. We already mentioned that diabetes can be overwhelming. Just breaking it down into smaller, more manageable parts can help tremendously.

A little exercise:

William Miller and Steven Rollnick developed the following scale that is helpful to determine confidence and importance. Answer these questions:

1) *On a scale of 1 to 10 (with 10 being the highest), how important is it to manage my diabetes?* If your answer is not a ten, why is that? What would it take to get it closer to ten?

2) *On a scale of 1 to 10 (with 10 being the highest), how confident am I that I can manage my diabetes?*

If your answer is not a ten, why is that? What would it take to get it closer to ten?

Take a moment and give yourself credit for all that you do: diabetes management tasks (whichever ones you might be doing), going to work, raising a family, or just getting up each morning and taking breaths. Pat yourself on the back for your accomplishments no matter how large or small. Then decide what you need to do next: what is most important and how can you make it happen? If you need to be inspired to take care of your diabetes, achieve a goal, or just get out of a slump, I strongly recommend reading *The Gift of Fire* by Dan Caro. Better yet, if you can hear him speak live, do it! This is a man who was burned on over 80% of his body at age two. He tells how he has overcome adversity – again and again – and achieved his goals. You can too!

Confidence is critical. You may have heard the quote, *"If you can imagine it, you can achieve it; if you can dream it, you can become it"* (William Arthur Ward). I believe this is true, and I equate that to believing in yourself. I also think it is pretty hard to achieve something that you don't believe in. And now I'm back to attitude. Believing in yourself and your ability to manage your diabetes and live a healthy, productive life is a healthy, positive attitude. Go grab it!

Sometimes we just have to be distracted to get our thoughts (and hands) off of food. One thing you can do is make a list of activities for when you are thinking about eating, but you don't want to. Just as the quote at the beginning of the chapter says, you can do something else to avoid eating extra, unwanted calories. Some ideas include crafts, phoning a friend, writing, reading a book/magazine, playing a game of solitaire, sudoku or a crossword puzzle (you can play a game with someone else if they are available and willing), going for a walk, listening to music, taking a nap, playing with your pet, making a list, cleaning, gardening, scrapbooking, laundry – whatever works for you!

A little exercise:

Make your own list of things to do when you need to be distracted from food:

_____

_____

_____

_____

_____

_____

_____

_____

_____

Health Beliefs

People have different beliefs about their health. These beliefs come from different sources – perhaps someone's parents instilled in them certain beliefs about health, or perhaps a past experience molded someone's beliefs. Some health beliefs are based on cultural beliefs. Understanding your beliefs about your health can help you figure out why you do the things you do with regard to your health. For instance, if you believe that you are going to get dreaded diabetes-related complications and die, you might have unconsciously decided not to bother taking care of yourself. I worked with a patient who needed to start insulin, and insisted she would not have anything to do with needles. It turned out this patient's husband had been very sick and died after a lot of intervention from the health care system. This woman was able to talk about how she felt the "system" was responsible for her husband's death, so she wanted nothing to do with it. She clearly stated that she would not go near the hospital again and the next time any health care folks would see her she'd be dead. This is an example of how what we believe about health can affect our willingness to take care of ourselves. Looking further into why you believe what you do about your health can help you understand and perhaps adjust some of those beliefs. Think about how your health beliefs affect where you are now and where you will be in 5, 10, 20 years or more!

Another way to look at your health beliefs is to think about threats to your health. What do you consider a threat to your health? How likely is that threat to affect you? How serious is the threat and how motivated are you to avoid the threat? Several years ago I had a scare with my eyes. I had an ophthalmologist tell me I needed an angiogram (where they inject dye into your vein and then watch it go through the vessels of your eyes, looking for leakage). I had so many plans that included the use of my eyes, and I could not afford to not be able to see! I had a wonderful nurse practitioner at the time who inspired me to fight eye disease with my attitude. She told me to "carry my flame" and say, "Complications (eye disease) will not happen to me" (or something like that). Over the years I began visualizing healthy eyes and adjusting my attitude to one of strength, not fear. Some of the plans I had at the time (getting my PhD in Nursing, getting married, having kids) have happened and some are still to come, and my eyes are stable.

A little exercise:

Write down your negative health beliefs and ideas for how you might work on changing each belief.

Health Belief:

_____

Change:

_____

Health Belief:

_____

Change:

_____

Health Belief:

_____

Change:

_____

On the other hand, health beliefs can be positive and lead to good habits. I believe strongly that my attitude determines my health outcomes. Your negative health beliefs – or any beliefs, for that matter – limit you and hold you back. You can choose to change those beliefs and make them positive.

A little exercise:

Write down your positive health beliefs and the positive outcomes they will deliver.

Health belief:

_____

Positive outcome:

_____

Health belief:

_____

Positive outcome:

_____

Health belief:

_____

Positive outcome:

_____

A little exercise:

Write your mantra. Make it a positive statement that you can repeat in your head that will help you move forward and take care of yourself. Here's mine: *I am healthy and whole.*

Here's yours:

_____

_____

Turn Guilt into Motivation

If you have diabetes, it's not your fault. There are many factors that played a role in your getting diabetes, including family history. Perhaps you feel that you could be doing things differently - eating less or making healthier choices. Women with gestational diabetes often experience guilt - they feel they have hurt their baby. Guilt is a common part of diabetes, but it doesn't have to be. You are not at fault, and it doesn't serve any purpose to dwell on the past or to succumb to guilt. Guilt doesn't help and it doesn't change anything. You are a good person, and you can move forward from where you are. Use the energy that you've been putting toward guilt and turn it into motivation instead. Use it to keep yourself on track (or get yourself back on track when you fall off). None of us - diabetes or not - is perfect. None of us does everything right all the time. Some of us are better at food choices than others. Some of us are better at exercising than others. Take this opportunity for a second chance. Cut yourself some slack. Give yourself credit for the teeny, tiny, baby steps you have taken (whatever they are). And then keep going. And if you mess up today or tomorrow or the next day, don't waste time or energy beating yourself up. Get back on track again and again – as many times as it takes until healthy choices become the norm and getting off track only happens every once in a while.

Courage does not always roar. Sometimes courage is the quiet voice at the end of the day saying, 'I will try again tomorrow.'

Mary Anne Radmacher

Chapter 11
Getting on with Life

Life needs to go on regardless of diabetes
Dad of a 6-year-old with type 1 diabetes

What was your experience like when you were first diagnosed with diabetes? Did your family/friends help you take it on? Or were you made to feel you had done something wrong or somehow failed? Were you scared, or did you know this is something you can handle? I feel very fortunate that my health care providers emphasized to my parents the importance of teaching me that I (we) could manage diabetes. That message still doesn't get across to many people when they are first diagnosed with diabetes. Your experience at diagnosis can truly have an impact on how you perceive – and take care of – your diabetes for the rest of your life.

You can do this.

Research has shown that people who received reassuring messages from health care professionals when they were diagnosed have a tendency to experience less diabetes distress and perform more effective diabetes self-management for up to five years after diagnosis (21). Unfortunately, there's no way to change the experience you had at diagnosis. You may have even been *mis*diagnosed. It is possible to do some work on your own or with the help of family, friends or a counselor, if you had a negative initial experience. You are not a bad person, and it is not your fault that you have diabetes. You have the strength and the ability to manage this disease.

You can do this.

If your child was recently diagnosed with diabetes, you may look at him/her and all you see is diabetes. Hopefully with time this will change. In my experience it can. If you are having difficulty with this, please consider talking to someone about it. I would suggest getting together with other parents to discuss how they handle diabetes and their child(ren). There are wonderful online resources, blogs, and networks for parents of children with diabetes. Surround yourself with positive role models who have a healthy attitude and a healthy approach toward living with diabetes. My father told me that the diabetes educator they met when I was diagnosed made it very clear that they (my parents) needed to show me that diabetes was not a big deal and that it was manageable. Pretty impressive for 1975, I think. We definitely know this is true today. Although diabetes *is* a big deal, taking it in stride can lead to better adjustment and success. And it's always good to have support along the diabetes journey. Whether you have diabetes yourself, or someone you care about has it, consider joining a support group. Everyone benefits from support.

Some of my closest friends – and definitely those I can talk to about anything – are my friends who have diabetes. Most of them I met at diabetes camp. It's comforting to be able to compare notes or just talk about every day stuff, and know that they completely understand the diabetes part. They know when to ask questions, and when not to. I can't emphasize enough the benefits of having people in your life who can relate to what you are experiencing. And they are out there – you just have to find them. Diabetes social networks are websites where you can "chat" with people who will understand you. If you can't find a suitable support group, consider starting a new one.

If someone were to ask me, "What were the biggest influences on your attitude toward diabetes?" I would answer: my parents and diabetes camp. My parents and camp were positive influences for different reasons. My parents always approached diabetes as something that was do-able and not a big deal. I don't remember them ever freaking out about diabetes or any part of its management. Maybe they did that when I wasn't around. My siblings and extended family never made a big deal of it either. My parents never gave me a hard time or questioned me about what I was doing. They trusted me, gave me a lot of responsibility and made me feel I was capable of handling it.

> **Tasty Morsel (of information):** For the first several years after I was diagnosed, my father took me to the hospital for quarterly blood tests. We would leave early in the morning for my "fasting" (blood test) and afterward we'd go out for breakfast. Dad would drive me to school and then pick me up a few hours later for my "non-fasting." This was our special time together, and despite being poked for the blood draws, I have great memories of hanging out with my dad. One danger in all this is that siblings might feel less attention is paid to them. Parents have to balance spending time with all their kids and not just focusing on the child with diabetes (or the diabetes itself).

As a camp counselor and then camp nurse, I learned a lot about diabetes. More importantly I met lifelong friends who also have diabetes. The responsibility of caring for younger children with diabetes along with the fun I had with my "compatriots" brought me to a new level of taking diabetes in stride. My camp friends are the ones I can call, email, or text whenever I need to talk about anything, and they understand how diabetes fits in. We don't even have to talk about diabetes – they just know. To each other we are people first, who happen to have diabetes.

Having this sort of support system gives me strength, confidence and reassurance. I attribute my healthy and positive attitude toward living with diabetes to having been "raised" in a healthy and positive diabetes environment.

I have also had some wonderful health care providers. When I was diagnosed I saw a pediatric endocrinologist for several years. When my parents' health insurance changed and we started going to an HMO (managed care), I saw a general pediatrician and then an internist once I turned eighteen. It wasn't until several years later that I began seeing an endocrinologist again, and then I typically met with the nurse practitioner. I have mentioned some of the insight she shared with me. Since relocating and my first pregnancy, I have been seeing an endocrinologist regularly. I prefer to work with a specialist, because he has so much experience with all aspects of diabetes and I appreciate his willingness to answer my questions and share whatever new information he has. It's also nice to see someone who works in a research center, since they know what is cutting edge and what is on the horizon in terms of diabetes treatment and gadgets.

It is very important for people with diabetes to find the right health care provider. Not everyone has the luxury of seeing a specialist. Some endocrinologists specialize in diabetes, and some endocrinologists see patients with other endocrinology disorders as well as diabetes. Primary care physicians, physician assistants and nurse practitioners can help you with your diabetes as well. Many of these health care professionals have a lot of diabetes experience. They read the latest research and attend conferences to stay current on diabetes medications and treatment options. Finding a provider who is a good fit for you makes it easier for you to talk openly with that person, ask questions and seek answers and support. Make sure you know what you are looking for in a health care provider and then go find that person. If you are working with someone who does not feel like a good fit (they don't meet your needs for whatever reason), it is perfectly ok to switch providers.

A little exercise:

Make a list of the qualities/characteristics that you are looking for in a health care provider:

_____

_____

_____

_____

_____

Be sure to write down your questions in between visits to your health care provider. Once you get to the office, it is easy to forget all your questions. If you have a little notebook with you, you can easily open it up and read/ask your questions. You can even write down the answers in your notebook. This is a great idea, especially because it's easy to hear one thing in the provider's office and then get home and either forget what was said or get it mixed up in your mind and come out with something totally different. If you have the answers in your notebook, you can refer back to what you wrote. Do not hesitate to ask for clarification if something your provider says doesn't make sense to you. It also helps to bring a friend or family member to your appointments. A second set of ears can help in "hearing" what the provider says. Later on, you can compare notes.

> **Tasty Morsel (of information)**: What is said and what we hear are sometimes two completely different things. Sometimes we are so stressed out in a health-related visit

that we don't hear clearly, and sometimes health care providers don't give us enough information or say it in a way that we understand. If you can't bring someone along, be sure to take notes. If you get home and realize you have questions, write them down and call or bring them with you the next time.

An endocrinologist is a medical doctor who spent extra time studying the endocrine system, which includes diabetes among other disorders. An internist is a medical doctor who specializes in Internal Medicine (basically, adult medicine). An endocrinologist is often an internist with extra training. A pediatric endocrinologist is an endocrinologist who specializes in pediatric endocrine disorders, including diabetes. A nurse practitioner (NP) is a registered nurse with an advanced degree (Masters or Doctorate), who manages all aspects of health for a population of people. Adult nurse practitioners take care of adults, pediatric nurse practitioners take care of children, and family nurse practitioners take care of both adults and children. Some NPs specialize in diabetes. A physician assistant or physician associate (PA) is a health care professional licensed to practice medicine under the supervision of a physician. Some PAs specialize in diabetes. A certified diabetes educator (CDE) is a health care professional who specializes in diabetes education and has met the requirements to take a certification exam. CDEs stay certified by taking continuing education and/or retaking the exam every five years. A board certified – advanced diabetes manager (BC-ADM) is a health care professional with an advanced degree who has met the requirements and passed an exam in advanced diabetes management.

Taking it off and keeping it off

We've discussed food a lot in this book. Overweight and obesity are a big part of diabetes. Many people with type 2 diabetes are overweight and many people with type 1 are too. Overweight and obesity are national problems for those without diabetes as well. Although this book is not about weight loss, many people can improve their health dramatically by losing weight. If you have diabetes and you want to lose weight, it is necessary to balance what you eat, what medications you take, and the activity you do. Work with your health care professional to figure these things out, so that you can be successful in your efforts. If you are experiencing consistent low blood glucose levels, you will have to eat additional calories, which defeats your purpose. Remember that the most effective weight loss programs focus on changing your lifestyle (making healthy choices), rather than going on a "diet."

The National Eating Disorder Association reported that dieters spend about $40 billion per year and 19 out of 20 people lose nothing but their money (22). The National Weight Control Registry studied people who lost 30 pounds or more and kept it off for at least one year. They found that these people were likely to follow these steps:

- Eat breakfast
- Monitor weight
- Count calories
- Choose sensible portions
- Exercise 60 minutes per day
- Watch less television (23)

If your weight goes down enough, your need for diabetes medication may go down too. Again, it is important to work closely with your health care provider to determine what changes you need to make.

When Diabetes Interferes with your Life

Is diabetes negatively affecting your work, school, social, or love life? Is it interfering with your productivity on a daily basis or often enough to get you down? Think about what is causing this to happen. Is it frequent low blood glucose levels or high blood glucose levels or fluctuating between the two? Do you find yourself overeating in response to stress, boredom, depression, or other things in your life? This list may seem obvious to some, but here's a reminder of the short-term, negative consequences that overeating can cause (at any point in the day):

- Food hangover: this is the way you feel after overeating.
- Fatigue
- Low productivity
- Difficulty getting out of bed or off the couch
- Lack of motivation to exercise
- Getting behind in work
- Decreased self-esteem

On the other hand, when blood glucose is in the target range, there is a tendency to feel clear. It's easier to be productive, which directly leads to feeling good about yourself.

A little exercise:

If you feel that your diabetes is chronically causing you frustration and lack of productivity, make a list of the contributing factors (overeating in response to X; lack of exercise because of X, etc.):

_____

_____

_____

_____

Now make a list of how you can deal with each of those situations, either on your own or with help (and include who/what would help you)

_____

_____

_____

_____

_____

One situation that can really interfere with your life is getting up in the middle of the night to check your blood glucose. If you are waking up low or high in the morning it makes sense to set an alarm and get up in the middle of the night to see what's happening. You might be getting too much insulin overnight (or not enough). Remember, high blood glucose in the morning can mean that you are not getting enough insulin, or that your long-acting insulin is running out too soon, or it can mean that you are having lows in the middle of the night and rebounding (see Chapter 8). But middle of the night blood glucose checks are not meant to become a routine part of your life. This is an interruption to your sleep and sleep is critical for everyone. If you are getting up to check overnight blood glucose levels on a loved one, this is not good for you or your loved one in the long-run. Again, an occasional check-in is fine, but if it starts to become routine, figure out a plan for doing without it (or using continuous glucose monitoring). Talk to your health care professional to see what you can change or adjust so that waking up in the middle of the night is not necessary.

Checking overnight blood glucose levels can be prompted by fear. There is often a lot of fear surrounding diabetes and diabetes management. This can be true for those with diabetes and for those who love people with diabetes. I can't even imagine how scary it would be to have a child with diabetes and send them off to a sleepover, or to school, or to camp. I often think about how fortunate I am not to have to worry about that with my kids. It's also frightening for the spouse of someone with diabetes who worries that they are low whenever they toss and turn or cry out in their sleep. What about when the loved one is not taking care of him/herself the way you wish they would?

For people with diabetes there is the constant fear of complications. There is the fear of hypoglycemia and what might happen if we are driving and have a low, or carrying our baby or running a marathon. We fear that high blood glucose will lower our immune defenses and expose us to illnesses that we don't want or have time for. We fear being asked about our diabetes, or perhaps not being asked. Perhaps we're afraid of negative assumptions people have about those with diabetes.

Fear does not have to consume us. We can manage this thing called diabetes and not let it take over our lives. The best way I can think of to do this is to stay in touch – with our bodies, with our emotions, with our needs, with our support systems, and with our health care providers. Remember that knowledge is power. The more we know and understand (and know how to handle), the less we have to fear. I have mentioned patients saying they were afraid of food, or afraid to eat. This is very common, and can be overcome with knowledge. If you understand how food affects your blood glucose, and what you can do to manage it, you don't have to fear food.

We can form networks with people like us – through diabetes camps and diabetes social networks. I once had a diabetes pen pal (for real – I "met" her through the American Diabetes Association's magazine, *Diabetes Forecast*, and we wrote letters to each other for years). There are online chat forums for people with diabetes, and although letter-writing may be a thing of the past, you can always email or text each other.

We can read books and ask questions. We can check our blood glucose levels routinely so that we know what is going on in our bodies and make conscious, healthy choices based on this information. We can give ourselves second, third, fourth, and so on, chances when we mess up or slip up. We can accept ourselves as the smart, creative, dedicated, hard-working people we are who are doing the best we can.

Everyone is different; what works for one person may not work for another. Some people discuss their diabetes openly, others tell no one or very few. The point of all this is to find not only what motivates you, but what works for you – in all aspects of diabetes and life. You are a unique person, and how you approach diabetes is or will be unique. If you are the parent of a child with diabetes, your job is to help guide them toward being healthy and independent. Show them how to work toward making their own diabetes (and life) choices. Success and failure are measured by our own standards/targets, not the standards of someone else. It is our responsibility to get and stay informed about our health. That way we can make informed decisions about our goals, standards and targets.

Chapter 12

For Those Who Care For Someone with Diabetes

If you care about someone with diabetes, it can be scary, overwhelming, frustrating and more. Maybe you are the person's caregiver or maybe just someone on the sidelines. Either way, you probably worry when you see them eat something you think they "can't eat." I hope that after reading this book you have a better understanding of diabetes. I am in no way saying that diabetes is easy, but I stand behind my belief that it is manageable. Following are some suggestions for more effective ways to care about/for someone with diabetes.

Trust them

Give your loved one the benefit of the doubt. Trust that they know what they are doing. Ask questions if you don't know or understand what they are doing. Ask in a way that still shows you trust them. And be trustworthy yourself. If you truly have reason to believe your loved one cannot be trusted, then start by communicating with them. Open dialogue is the best way to find out what's going on for your loved one.

Give them space

You may know how it feels to have someone breathing down your neck – whether that's a boss or a parent, it's just no fun. It goes hand-in-hand with trusting your loved one with diabetes. Don't hover (unless they ask you to)! Avoid sheltering, suffocating or nagging your loved one who has diabetes. Often these behaviors just lead to the one with diabetes rebelling, which might mean overeating or neglecting other diabetes management tasks.

Be a good communicator

Let your loved one know your concerns – in a kind way. Tell them that you want them to be around for a long time so you can

_____ (fill in the activities you would like to enjoy together). Ask them what you can do to help or support them in their diabetes management. If you have a concern or frustration that is diabetes-related, sit down and talk about it. Don't let it fester inside until you boil over!

My friend's husband has type 1 diabetes. In the past he would have a low blood glucose and become belligerent and refuse to treat the low. My friend communicated with her husband that it scared her when he was low. Her husband responded to her concern and together they came up with a plan. If she asks him to check his blood glucose, he does it.

Accept them

Your loved one has diabetes. This is an important part of them, but does not define them. Treat them the same as you would if they did not have diabetes. If you struggle with this concept, go back to the "be a good communicator" step and have a talk with them. Figure out what your struggle is and work through it.

Support them

You can support your loved one with diabetes in many different ways. You can exercise with them. Be their walking, running, swimming, etc., partner. Be their cheerleader and help them stay motivated to exercise routinely – you'll both benefit. You can also support them by respecting their needs in the food department. If your loved one has no self-control around certain food items, do them a favor and don't bring those items into the house. As inconvenient as it might be, keep them in your car or at your workplace. Yes, it would be nice if we could just not eat certain foods, but it's easier if some foods are not in the house.

Encourage them

Encouragement might be noticing if your loved one has lost weight, complimenting them on being active, making a healthy choice, or a healthy (delicious) meal they prepared. Or you could prepare a healthy, delicious meal for them. Other ways to encourage your loved one might be to send them to camp or to college.

A family friend was diagnosed with diabetes at age 18 – two weeks before the start of college. Her mother got an earful from all sorts of friends and family members, saying she should keep her daughter home and "watch" her. This friend sent her daughter to college, where she became independent in her diabetes management and did very well. I'm sure there were some scary moments for this mom, but she trusted her daughter, gave her space, supported her, and encouraged her. Maybe the scenario is different and it's not college but a trip or a job in a new location. Regardless, it's important to encourage your loved one to be independent.

I mentioned in the introduction that I often get phone calls from family members of people with diabetes. They want to know what kind of food to have in the house when their family member with diabetes visits. Hopefully you have already gathered from this book the answer to that question: ask the person with diabetes! Call your son-in-law, aunt, friend – whoever is coming to visit – and ask if there is anything special they'd like you to have on hand when they come to stay. Chances are they will say no (or they might want to do their own shopping), but in any case you'll be prepared.

When I first got married and moved away, my parents used to ask what foods and beverages I wanted them to buy when we were coming to visit. Eventually they knew to have (plain) Cheerios®, skim (fat-free) milk, and a few staples for the kids. My husband's beverage of choice always seems to change just when they get it down. Oh well. My grandfather always kept diet soda in the basement refrigerator for me, which was very thoughtful of him. Unfortunately, it would sometimes be there for years at a time and would taste awful by the time I drank it! As a result, I was a very early supporter of expiration dates on sodas.

You love someone with diabetes, and you wish they didn't have it. You wish they didn't have to poke, inject, take pills, or think about what they eat. You might even wish they were "normal." As hard as it might be, I encourage you to think of them as "normal" anyway, because diabetes is *their* normal. Remember that one's diabetes belongs to him or her. It's ok for you to be involved (within the boundaries you've set together), but you can't do it for them (at least not in most cases). It's ok to let go and it's ok to trust. From all of us with diabetes, thank you for your concern, your care, and your love. Just like the dad quoted at the beginning of Chapter 11 said, "Life needs to go on regardless of diabetes." That means your life too - now go take some time for yourself!

Epilogue

It is better to believe than to disbelieve, in so doing you bring everything to the realm of possibility. Albert Einstein

Now it's time for you to go out in the world and take care of yourself. Manage your diabetes. Make healthy choices. Have a great attitude. And it won't be easy all the time. There will be some good moments and some bad moments; some easy times and some hard times. Every moment, however, includes choices. You get to choose how you react, what you do, what you eat, how you feel. You get only one life: you don't get to decide how long it is, but you get to determine the quality of it.

Believe in yourself: you can do this. Whatever you are doing for your diabetes at this point, pat yourself on the back for it. It counts. If you are taking your medications routinely – good work! If you are checking your blood glucose (however often), good for you! If you are eating more vegetables, or watching portion sizes, or taking walks - nice job!

If you are doing nothing other than getting up each morning and breathing in and out – that's ok too. Now it's time to make a plan, set some goals and add something more to your diabetes routine. Instead of taking things away from yourself, *add* things such as vegetables, exercise, stress management skills or distraction techniques. Make peace with food; don't think of food as the enemy. Try being friends with food. You can eat anything and you are in charge of the choices you make. Find healthy ways to make healthy food delicious. You can do this.

When you have bad days or set-backs, give yourself a break and move on. Find ways to laugh about it and stay positive. Figure out how your mindset or attitude might be limiting you and work to turn that around. Remember that blood glucose levels are just numbers: information to help you make your next choice. Consider finding others who understand what you are experiencing. There are many support groups and resources available for people who have diabetes. The internet is loaded with diabetes social networks and blogs. Blogging is a great way to meet others, compare experiences, and even stay anonymous if you like your privacy. If you are really motivated, you can always start your own support group, organization, team, website or blog. You could even write a book!

Throughout this book I have provided some "exercises" to do on your own. If you have never been fond of doing this sort of thing (writing down goals), I urge you to give it a try now. You never know. I've also made several suggestions for additional reading. Those books - plus a couple extra - are all listed in the Appendix. I have decided not to provide a list of social networks and blogs, however, because there are so many and I wouldn't want to leave any out. More importantly, new social networks and blogs are being created all the time. Take some time to search the Internet for "diabetes social networks" and "diabetes blogs." You will be amazed at what you find. There are even weekly live chats. Remember that you may or may not have something in common with the author of a particular site. If not, keep looking.

Please join me in the blogosphere, by checking out www.janekdickinson.com. I'd love to hear from you. Also, this book is just as much for those without diabetes as it is for those with diabetes. Please feel free to share it with friends and family, so they too can understand that diabetes management is all about choices, attitude, and ownership. Encourage them to visit some diabetes blogs and talk openly about what you (and they) find there.

Final Thoughts

My father has been giving me the annual American Diabetes Association "gift of hope" Christmas ornament every year since the program started in 1986. At Christmastime I hang all of them in a big window in our kitchen. My daughter once asked me, "Mom, how long is Papa going to keep giving you these ornaments?" And I answered, "Until there is a cure for diabetes and we don't need to hope for it anymore." As long as I can remember, the cure for diabetes has been "about five years away."

I'll be honest; I do believe diabetes will be cured someday. I don't know if it will be in my lifetime. I do, however, believe a prevention for diabetes could be discovered and even perfected in my lifetime. I've been known to say that "I don't live for a cure," and this is true. I live for today and I accept that diabetes is part of it. I understand that parents, friends, and family of those with diabetes might "live for a cure" because they want to see their loved one free from the burden of diabetes. However, I'm more focused on living my life – and taking care of myself so I can live my life fully – than worrying about the future.

With type 1 diabetes, a cure is pretty straight forward: it will require finding a way for us to permanently regain the ability to produce insulin. There is a continuous debate about whether type 2 diabetes can be "cured." Some people say that type 2 diabetes can be in "remission" if someone keeps their blood glucose level in the normal range all the time. It's important to remember that even with normal blood glucose levels, you still have diabetes. If you were to go back to your old eating habits and not exercising, your blood glucose readings would creep right back up.

Every once in a while I think about a world without diabetes. I am very grateful to the smart people who are working hard to cure diabetes. And I would be ok with being put out of work, by the way. It would certainly be fun to go back to camp ("for kids who used to have diabetes") and hang out, maybe reminisce for a while. It would be nice not to worry about complications or doing all the daily tasks of diabetes management. It would be extremely strange to eat a meal without checking my blood glucose or taking insulin first, but I'm quite sure I could get used to it! My hope, once there is a cure, is that we will all remember and continue to practice the healthy habits we developed while managing diabetes.

If there is anything positive about living with diabetes it's that I have learned to manage stress, exercise, and make healthy food choices most of the time. I have a greater appreciation for my health and my body: my eyes, kidneys, nerves, heart, blood vessels, joints – *the whole thing*. I am aware of how I treat my body and I strive to take good care of it (don't always succeed, but strive). Because of diabetes I am aware of how I define quality of life, what is important to me, and what my priorities are. And I make it a point to accomplish all of it. Through living with diabetes I have learned the power of attitude and balance in all things. I do not let diabetes run my life, yet I have a healthy respect toward it. And that is my choice.

Appendix

Jane's Recommended Reading List:

The Sugarless Plum	Zippora Karz
The Discovery of Insulin	Michael Bliss
Exchange Lists for Diabetes	American Diabetes Association
The Complete Guide to Carbohydrate Counting	Hope Warshaw and Karmeen Kulkarni
Intuitive Eating	Evelyn Tribole and Elyse Resch
The Art and Science of Low Carbohydrate Living	Jeff Volek and Stephen Phinney
Stretching	Bob Anderson
The Gift of Fire	Dan Caro
Raising Lazarus	Robert Pensack and Dwight Williams
When You're a Parent with Diabetes	Kathryn Palmer
Succeed: How We Can Reach Our Goals	Heidi Grant Halvorson
Eat Out, Eat Right	Hope Warshaw
Guide to Healthy Restaurant Eating	Hope Warshaw
365 Daily Meditations For People With Diabetes	Catherine Feste
The Power of Visualization	Lee Pulos
Breakthrough	Thea Cooper
Mindless Eating	Brian Wansink

There are so many great books that it's hard to make a list. These are just some to get you started. Please visit me in the Diabetes Online Community at www.janekdickinson.com.

References

Here is a list of articles to support sections from my book. The numbers correspond to the numbers in the book. In many cases I have chosen to cite non-scholarly references because I think they are often easier to read and understand. If you are looking for something more scientific, the research articles are often cited in these articles. You are also welcome to visit me at my website (www.janekdickinson.com), and I can help you find something.

1. Centers for Disease Control and Prevention (2011). National Diabetes Fact Sheet. Retrieved from
http://www.cdc.gov/diabetes/pubs/pdf/ndfs_2011.pdf

2. Pyhtila, H. (2007). Thrifty Genes. Retrieved from
http://www.genomebc.ca/education/articles/thrifty-genes/

3. Hill, L.W. (1916). The Starvation Treatment of Diabetes. Retrieved from http://www.gutenberg.org/files/26058/26058-h/26058-h.htm

4. Franz, M.J., Bantle, J.P., Beebe, C.A., Brunzell, J.D., Chiasson, J-L., Garg, A., Holzmeister, L.A., et al. (2002). Evidence-Based Nutrition Principles and Recommendations for the Treatment and Prevention of Diabetes and Related Complications. Retrieved from
http://care.diabetesjournals.org/content/25/1/148.full

5. Reuters (2011). Is the Apple or Pear-Shaped Body Type More Dangerous? Retrieved from http://www.huffingtonpost.com/2011/03/11/apple-pear-shaped_n_834575.html

6. Hensrud, D. (2010). Weight Loss. Retrieved from http://www.mayoclinic.com/health/low-fat-vs-low-carb/MY01446/

7. Mayo Clinic Staff (2011). Alcohol Use: If you drink, keep it moderate. Retrieved from http://www.mayoclinic.com/health/alcohol/SC00024

8. Lipman, R. (2009). Weight Loss and Portion Control - More important than exercising. Retrieved from http://ezinearticles.com/?Weight-Loss-and-Portion-Control---More-Important-Than-Exercising&id=3425391

9. Parker-Pope, T. (2007). The Risks and Rewards of Skipping Meals. Retrieved from http://well.blogs.nytimes.com/2007/12/26/the-risks-and-rewards-of-skipping-meals/

10. Healy, M. (2011). Hormones Feed Hunger After Weight Loss, Researchers Find. Retrieved from http://www.columbian.com/news/2011/oct/27/hormones-feed-hunger-after-weight-loss-researchers/

11. Blair, S. & Brodney, S. (1999). Effects of Physical Inactivity and Obesity on Morbitidy and Mortality: Current evidence and research issues. Retrieved from http://www.uoguelph.ca/hhns/grad/pdf_grad/HBNS6710W08BlairandBrodney.pdf

12. Hendrick, B. (2010). Exercise Helps You Sleep. Retrieved from http://www.webmd.com/sleep-disorders/news/20100917/exercise-helps-you-sleep

13. Mayo Clinic Staff (2010). Exercise Helps Ease Arthritis Pain and Stiffness. Retrieved from http://www.mayoclinic.com/health/arthritis/AR00009/

14. National Institutes of Diabetes and Digestive and Kidney Diseases - National Diabetes Information Clearinghouse (2012). The A1C Test and Diabetes. Retrieved from http://diabetes.niddk.nih.gov/dm/pubs/A1CTest/#15

15. National Institutes of Diabetes and Digestive and Kidney Diseases - National Diabetes Information Clearinghouse (2012). DCCT and EDIC: The Diabetes Control and Complications Trial and Follow-Up Study. Retrieved from http://diabetes.niddk.nih.gov/dm/pubs/control/

16. Council for the Advancement of Diabetes Research and Education (2011). Treatment Guidelines: A1C Recommendations. Retrieved from http://www.cadre-diabetes.org/r_treatment_guidelines.asp

17. Monnier, L. & Collette, C. (2006). Contributions of fasting and postprandial plasma glucose increments to the overall diurnal hyperglycemia of type 2 diabetic patients: variations with increasing levels of HbA(1c). Retrieved from
http://www.ncbi.nlm.nih.gov/pubmed/16627379

18. EASD Annual Meeting (2010). One in Three Patients Fail to Take Insulin as Prescribed, Survey Says. Retrieved from
http://www.healio.com/endocrinology/diabetes/news/online/%7B7d4732
08-86d8-4b57-bf8c-85d3e589ab59%7D/one-in-three-patients-fail-to-take-insulin-as-prescribed-survey-says

19. Polonsky, W. & Jackson R. (2004). What's so Tough About Taking Insulin? Addressing the Problem of Psychological Insulin Resistance in Type 2 Diabetes. Retrieved from
http://clinical.diabetesjournals.org/content/22/3/147.full

20. Gavard, J., Lustman, P. & Clouse, R. (1993). Prevalence of Depression in Adults with Diabetes. Retrieved from
http://care.diabetesjournals.org/content/16/8/1167.full.pdf+html

21. Polonsky, W., Fisher, L., Guzman, S., Sieber, W., Philis-Tsimikas, A. & Edelman, S. (2010). Are Patients' Initial Experiences at the Diagnosis of Type 2 Diabetes Associated with Attitudes and Self-management Over Time? Retrieved from
http://tde.sagepub.com/content/36/5/828

22. McLaughlin, A. (2011). Preoccupation with Food and Weight Loss. Retrieved from http://www.livestrong.com/article/255157-preoccupation-with-food-weight-loss/

23. The National Weight Control Registry (No Date). NWCR Facts. Retrieved from http://www.nwcr.ws/Research/default.htm

Acknowledgements

I am grateful to the many people who helped me get this project from thoughts to words to a full-fledged book. The idea originated at a small town hospital in Colorado; Carol Mahoney was a fellow champion of the philosophy that "people with diabetes can eat anything." Cece Carsky took up the cause, gave me further motivation to write, and provided invaluable feedback. My husband, Randall Hannaway, has supported my writing/publishing efforts all along the way. My parents, sister and brother answered questions and asked how things were going, without ever pressuring or doubting. My kids have been enthusiastic and energetic supporters for way too long. Deirdre Madden listened to my challenges and concerns during numerous phone calls. Jill Murphy Long was an early cheerleader, who taught me a lot about writing and publishing. The Women in Networking (WIN) Steamboat group gave me courage and encouragement. Todd Musselman held me to the fire. Tina Kyprios, David Street, Christine McKelvie, Jay Freschi, Kimberley Krapek, and Dana Cossey generously gave their time to read my book at various stages and provided helpful feedback. Countless friends cheered me on. The Diabetes Online Community gave me inspiration and hope. A heartfelt thank you to all of you!

About the Author

Jane K. Dickinson has been living with diabetes since 1975, and helping others live with diabetes since 1995. Jane is a registered nurse and certified diabetes educator. She earned her Bachelor of Arts in Biology from St. Olaf College, her Master of Science in Nursing from Yale University and her PhD in Nursing from the University of Connecticut.

In 2000, Jane developed the Yampa Valley Medical Center's Diabetes Education Program in Steamboat Springs, Colorado, which she managed until 2011. She continues working with diabetes patients through this local program. Before moving to Colorado, Jane was the Director of Clinical Services and Education for The Barton Center for Diabetes Education in North Oxford, Massachusetts.

In March of 2011, Jane became the Program Coordinator/Faculty for the Diabetes Education and Management Masters Program at Teachers College Columbia University (www.tc.edu/diabetes).

Jane's blog at www.janekdickinson.com provides straight-forward information about diabetes mixed with stories from Jane's personal and professional experiences. Jane is also connected with the Diabetes Online Community through Twitter, Facebook, LinkedIn, and tudiabetes.org. Jane lives in Steamboat Springs, Colorado, with her husband and two children.

About the Cover Designer

Erin O'Neill Argueta, who designed the book cover, has been living with type 1 diabetes for 40 years. Erin, who is a wife and mother of two, is a freelance card designer and mixed media artist who always believed she was born with three unique genetic characteristics: a creative gene, an adventurous gene and one dysfunctional gene that showed itself when she turned two. Erin uses her art as a means to calm herself and stay focused. Visit Erin's blog at www.edonadesigns.blogspot.com

About the Scale on the Cover

The scale on the cover is a Landers, Frary & Clark from New Britain, Connecticut. The scale is special to the author because it belonged to her grandmother; however, Jane has never weighed any food on it. To Jane, scales are a reminder to seek balance in all parts of her life.

www.ingramcontent.com/pod-product-compliance
Lightning Source LLC
Chambersburg PA
CBHW072124270326
41931CB00010B/1661

* 9 7 8 0 9 8 8 9 3 4 2 0 7 *